Department of Health and Social Security

Report on Health and Social Subjects

26

REPORT ON CONFIDENTIAL ENQUIRIES INTO MATERNAL DEATHS IN ENGLAND AND WALES 1976 – 1978

John Tomkinson CBE MB ChB FRCS FRCOG
Alexander Turnbull CBE MD ChB FRCOG
Sir Gordon Robson CBE MB ChB FRCS FFARCS
Ian Dawson MD FRCP FRC Path
Elizabeth Cloake MB BS DPH MFCM
A M Adelstein MD DPH FRCP FFCM
John Ashley MB ChB FFCM

London

Her Majesty's Stationery Office

ISBN 0 11 320814 6

Preface

This is the ninth report in the series on maternal deaths. Since 1967 – 69 these reports have been published in the series 'Reports on Health and Social Subjects' produced under the auspices of the Department of Health and Social Security, and this is number 26 in this series. The main authors of the ninth report on the Confidential Enquiries into Maternal Deaths are the Department's Consultant Advisers in Obstetrics and Gynaecology, Mr J S Tomkinson and Professor A C Turnbull, the Consultant Adviser in Anaesthetics Professor Sir Gordon Robson and the Consultant Adviser in Histopathology Professor I M P Dawson. Professor V R Tindall who was appointed as a Consultant Adviser in Obstetrics and Gynaecology in 1981 has also given invaluable assistance with the preparation of the report. They have had the help of Dr A M Adelstein and Dr J Ashley and the staff of the Medical Statistics Unit of the Office of Population, Censuses and Surveys, Dr Elizabeth Cloake in the Department of Health and Social Security and Dr Marie Richards in the Welsh Office. The regional assessors in obstetrics, whose names are given in Appendix C of the report have met under the chairmanship of Dr Gillian Ford, Deputy Chief Medical Officer, to discuss the contents of the report with the authors. The regional assessors in anaesthetics, although they did not meet centrally, were all consulted on the content of the chapter on deaths associated with anaesthesia. The final assessments therefore take account of the views expressed by all the assessors, and these have been co-ordinated by the named authors to produce a report generally acceptable to all those who contributed.

With the publication of this report the enquiry has now covered a period of 27 years. The present report includes 227 deaths directly due to pregnancy and childbirth and 200 due to associated causes. This report covers over 99% of all the known true obstetric deaths and only one such death was not reported to the enquiry. The maternal mortality rate (excluding abortion) during the triennium was 11.9 per 100,000 total births. The differences between the rates in the Regions showed considerable variation from 5.4 in the Wessex Region to 18.0 in the North East Thames Region. The proportion of true obstetric deaths (excluding deaths from abortion and ectopic pregnancy) which had one or more avoidable factors was 59% compared with 57.8% in 1973 – 75.

In several respects the main findings of the present report were very similar to those in 1973 – 75. The considerable improvements recorded in 1973 – 75 compared with 1970 – 72 were maintained, particularly in the reduced numbers of deaths from abortion and sepsis. However, the total number of true obstetric deaths, the maternal mortality rate and the percentage of deaths with avoidable factors remained comparatively unchanged. The improvement shown in 1976 – 78 in the reduction of the number of deaths from hypertensive diseases of pregnancy, in which the death rate fell substantially for the first time since 1967 – 69, was counter-balanced by a rise in the death rates from pulmonary embolism and haemorrhage.

As the total number of maternal deaths falls it becomes more difficult to achieve further reductions. The authors have particularly highlighted the deaths from haemorrhage in this report. Haemorrhage was found to have been a major factor in 76 of the 227 cases of true maternal death when its contribution to other named causes such as rupture of the uterus and ectopic pregnancy were taken into account. They have strongly recommended that each obstetric unit should have its own agreed procedure for the treatment of catastrophic haemorrhage.

As in previous reports emphasis has been placed on death rates per million maternities for individual cause of death so that comparisons between triennia can continue to be made despite the variations in the birth rate. However, in this report a new technique has been introduced to compare the number of deaths from individual causes during the 1976 – 78 triennium with those occurring in previous years, usually the period 1967 – 75. The number of 'expected' deaths on the basis of age and parity has been compared with the number of 'actual' deaths. The method used is described in Chapter I, and is first shown in Tables 2.2 and 2.3.

Another new feature of this report is the subdivision of the 200 deaths associated with pregnancy into *indirect* maternal deaths (97) and *fortuitous* deaths (103). This follows the International recommendations on maternal deaths, and these definitions are explained in Chapter I.

The importance of accurate diagnosis of the cause of death was emphasized in the last report. Early in 1980 the other authors were joined by a Central Assessor in Pathology, Professor Dawson, who has not only given advice on individual case reports but has also contributed a new chapter on post mortem examinations in cases of maternal death, Chapter 15. (In March 1981 Regional Assessors in Pathology were also appointed, too late to effect the present report, but their contribution will begin to be apparent in the cases for the 1979 – 81 report, which are still being assessed.)

I would like to thank the obstetricians, anaesthetists, pathologists, general practitioners, area medical officers, coroners and midwives who have so willingly made their detailed contributions to the individual reports. I am particularly indebted to the authors, the regional assessors and others who have undertaken the work of collating, analysing and commenting upon them.

This series of reports was one of the first examples of medical monitoring in any branch of medicine. Over the years it has gained both a national and international reputation. It has set the pattern for confidential enquiries into other fields of practice. I am sure that this, the original Confidential Enquiry still has much of value to contribute both now and in the future to the practice of obstetrics.

H YELLOWLEES
Chief Medical Officer
July, 1982

Contents

1. Introduction

The pattern of fertility 1976 – 1978

This is the ninth report of the series on confidential enquiries into maternal deaths and covers the three years 1976, 1977 and 1978. The period includes the year 1977 in which was recorded the lowest birth rate (11.7 per 1,000) in England and Wales since the start of civil registration in 1837 (Table 1.1).

Table 1.1: *Numbers of births and related death rates 1952 – 1978, England and Wales*

Year	Total births (live and still) in England and Wales	Births rate per 1,000 home population	Maternal mortality (excluding abortions) per 1,000 total births	Stillbirths (fetal deaths at 28 weeks or more of gestation) per 1,000 total births	Early neonatal mortality (deaths under 1 week) per 1,000 live births	Perinatal mortality (stillbirths and deaths under 1 week) per 1,000 total births
1952	689,371	15.7	0.54	22.7	15.2	37.5
1953	700,053	15.9	0.60	22.4	14.8	36.9
1954	689,851	15.6	0.54	23.5	14.9	38.1
1955	683,640	15.4	0.50	23.2	14.6	37.4
1956	716,740	16.0	0.42	22.9	14.2	36.7
1957	739,996	16.5	0.37	22.5	14.1	36.2
1958	757,003	16.8	0.35	21.5	13.8	35.0
1959	764,402	16.8	0.32	20.8	13.6	34.1
1960	800,824	17.5	0.31	19.8	13.3	32.8
1961	827,008	17.9	0.27	19.0	13.3	32.0
1962	884,200	18.3	0.28	18.1	13.0	30.8
1963	869,044	18.5	0.22	17.2	12.3	29.3
1964	890,518	18.8	0.20	16.3	12.0	28.2
1965	876,566	18.4	0.19	15.8	11.3	26.9
1966	863,066	18.0	0.20	15.3	11.1	26.3
1967	844,692	17.5	0.16	14.8	10.7	25.4
1968	831,120	17.1	0.18	14.3	10.6	24.7
1969	808,192	16.6	0.15	13.2	10.3	23.4
1970	794,831	16.2	0.14	13.0	10.6	23.5
1971	793,054	16.2	0.13	12.5	9.9	22.3
1972	734,239	15.0	0.12	12.0	9.8	21.7
1973	683,889	13.9	0.11	11.6	9.5	21.0
1974	647,060	13.2	0.11	11.1	9.4	20.4
1975	609,740	12.4	0.11	10.3	9.1	19.3
1976	589,979	12.0	0.12	9.7	8.1	17.7
1977	574,664	11.7	0.12	9.4	7.6	17.0
1978	601,526	12.2	0.10	8.5	7.1	15.5

Source: OPCS 1980a 1980b

From the last quarter of 1977 the numbers of births rose steadily in comparison with the corresponding quarters of previous years. Although the popu-

1

lation of women aged 15 – 44 continued to rise over the triennium, the increase in the number of live births in 1978 was attributable to an increased rate of childbearing (Table 1.2).

Table 1.2: *Total birth (live and still) rate per 1,000 home population, 1975 – 1979*

Year	Quarter				
	March	June	September	December	Annual
1975	12.9	12.9	12.4	11.4	12.4
1976	12.5	12.4	12.0	11.0	12.0
1977	11.7	12.0	12.0	11.2	11.7
1978	11.9	12.3	12.6	12.2	12.2
1979	13.0	13.5	13.2	12.6	13.1

The fertility rate in 1978 at 60.7 live births per 1,000 women aged 15 – 44 was over 3 per cent higher than in the previous year, when it was 58.7 and virtually identical with the rate two years earlier (60.9). The greatest increase in fertility rates between 1977 and 1978 was for women aged 30 – 39 (8 per cent). In contrast there was no change in the rate for women aged under 20. The rise in the fertility rate first became noticeable for the older women and spread progressively down the age-groups over time. It was evident at ages 30 – 34 in the first quarter of 1977, followed by the 25 – 29 age-group during the third quarter and eventually the under 25's by the last quarter of 1977.

Although all the Social Classes showed a rise in legitimate live births between 1977 and 1978, for Social Classes I and II (Professional and Technical) it was also noticeable one year previously (Table 1.3). Interestingly, the decline between 1970 and 1976 had been smaller in Classes I and II than in other classes.

Table 1.3: *Estimated legitimate live births by social class of father, England and Wales, 1970 to 1978*

Thousands

	Social Class				Non-manual	Manual	Total (inc others)
	I + II	IIIN	IIIM	IV and V			
1970	148.2	76.2	300.8	167.7	224.4	468.8	719.7
1971	154.7	75.3	297.9	160.1	229.9	458.0	717.5
1972	151.6	71.3	272.1	141.4	222.9	413.5	662.9
1973	148.1	64.5	245.8	130.7	212.6	376.5	617.9
1974	146.1	59.6	232.5	120.4	205.8	352.9	583.4
1975	141.6	57.0	214.1	111.8	198.6	325.9	548.6
1976	140.8	55.5	204.6	110.2	196.3	314.8	530.5
1977	142.3	53.2	193.4	106.6	195.5	300.0	513.9
1978	150.5	54.6	202.1	111.5	205.1	313.7	535.8

Source: OPCS 1980a

There has also been a recent rise in the number and proportion of legitimate live births to mothers whose birthplace was outside the United Kingdom

(Table 1.4). New Commonwealth 'immigrants', and those from Pakistan account for a significant part of this rise.

During the triennium the maternal mortality rate was effectively stationary but the perinatal mortality rate continued to fall substantially (see again Table 1.1 and Figure 1A).

Table 1.4: *Livebirths in England and Wales by birthplace of mother, 1976 – 1978*

Birthplace of mother	Number of live births (thousands)			Percentage of all live births		
	1976	1977	1978	1976	1977	1978
Total	584.3	569.3	569.4	100.0	100.0	100.0
United Kingdom	511.2	494.5	517.8	87.5	86.9	86.8
Total outside UK	72.4	74.2	78.1	12.4	13.0	13.1
Irish Republic	11.4	10.4	9.8	2.0	1.8	1.6
Australia, Canada, New Zealand	2.1	2.2	2.2	0.4	0.4	0.4
New Commonwealth	33.8	34.8	36.8	5.8	6.1	6.2
Bangladesh, India	13.5	13.9	14.2	2.3	2.4	2.4
Africa	6.7	7.5	8.3	1.1	1.3	1.4
West Indies	7.2	6.9	7.1	1.2	1.2	1.2
Malta, Gibraltar, Cyprus	2.8	2.7	2.9	0.5	0.5	0.5
Remainder of New Commonwealth	3.7	3.8	4.3	0.6	0.7	0.4
Pakistan	8.2	9.5	11.2	1.4	1.7	1.9
Other Foreign	16.9	17.3	18.2	2.9	3.0	3.0
Not Stated	0.7	0.6	0.5	0.1	0.1	0.1

Source: OPCS 1980a

During the previous triennium there had been a fall in legal terminations of pregnancy to residents of England and Wales from a peak in 1973 (OPCS, 1980c). In the period under review the annual numbers again rose to reach in 1978, a level similar to that of five years earlier (Table 1.5); of course the birth rate also rose during 1978.

Table 1.5: *Legal abortions, 1968 – 1978, residents in England and Wales*

Year	Number
1968 (8 months)	22,332
1969	49,829
1970	75,962
1971	94,570
1972	108,565
1973	110,568
1974	109,445
1975	106,224
1976	101,912
1977	102,677
1978	111,851

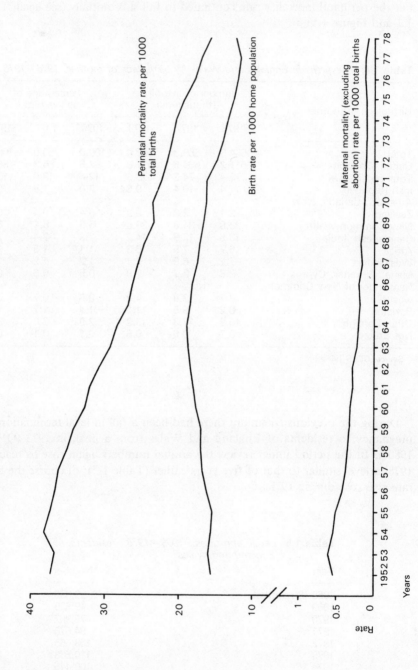

Figure 1A Birth rate per 1000 home population, perinatal mortality rate per 1000 total births and maternal mortality (excluding abortion) rate per 1000 total births 1952-1978

Perinatal mortality rate per 1000 total births

Birth rate per 1000 home population

Maternal mortality (excluding abortion) rate per 1000 total births

Rate

Years

4

Method of the enquiry

As in the last Report (DHSS, 1979) in the case of a known, or suspected, maternal death an enquiry was initiated by the Area Medical Officer (AMO) of the area in which the woman concerned was usually resident. An enquiry form (MCW 97) was sent for completion to all the health staff who had been concerned in the care of the woman, including general practitioners, midwives, health visitors, community physicians, consultant obstetricians and any other relevant staff at any hospital involved. Every possible attempt was made to obtain details of a post mortem examination including histology.

When all the available local information about the death had been collected the AMO forwarded the form to the appropriate regional assessor, a senior consultant obstetrician. In addition an anaesthetic assessor reviewed the enquiry forms of women who had received an anaesthetic. Both assessors added their comments and analysis, identified the cause or causes of death and assessed whether or not there had been avoidable factors in the sequence of events associated with the death.

The form was then sent to the Chief Medical Officer of the Department of Health and Social Security (DHSS) where it was matched with an extract from the appropriate death certificate. Of the 428 deaths known to the Enquiry 424 (99 per cent) had an MCW 97 form completed; three of the remaining four cases were among the 19 deaths reported by Coroners (see Appendix B) and in only one case was the information restricted to that on a death certificate mentioning pregnancy as a contributory cause of death.(Table 1.6). Three of these were associated deaths and one was a true death.

Table 1.6: *Sources of information about maternal deaths, 1976 – 1978*

	Deaths reported by Coroners to DHSS	Deaths not reported by Coroners	Total
Confidential Enquiry Form (MCW 97)	16	408	424
No Confidential Enquiry Form	3	1*	4
Total	19	409	428

* with death certificate mentioning pregnancy

It is again strongly emphasized that strict confidentiality is observed at all stages and the identity of the patient is also eradicated. The record of the opinions of the assessors cannot be related to a named individual, and after preparation of the report all MCW 97 forms are destroyed.

The Department's consultant advisers in Obstetrics and Gynaecology together with the consultant advisers in Anaesthetics and Histopathology (see Chapter 15) have reviewed all the available recorded facts about each case and acted as final arbiters identifying contributory causes and assessing the many factors that may have led to death.

It is possible that avoidance of some particular factor in an individual case would have resulted in the mother remaining alive. As in previous reports the assessors attempted, after considering the circumstances of each case, to decide whether an alternative choice of action by any individual would have prevented or reduced the likelihood of death. The factors were classified as 'avoidable', where there was a departure from generally accepted standards of satisfactory care during the triennium. The status of the person(s) responsible including the patient was indicated.

Throughout the 27 years history of these confidential enquiries the presence of avoidable factors has been recorded; there has been a rise in the generally accepted standards of satisfactory care over the same period, which may have been partly as a consequence of the publication of these reports. It is therefore not surprising to find that the proportion of deaths associated with avoidable factors has not decreased as have the absolute numbers of deaths and the mortality rates. Indeed the entry of new consultant advisers in obstetrics and anaesthetics will bring fresh viewpoints and alter standards. In this report most of the avoidable factors concern failure to provide appropriate care. Failure by medical staff to provide, or by patients to accept, advice about contraception, sterilization or termination of pregnancy has never been classed as an avoidable factor although there is a strong view that this should be considered in future. As in previous reports an illegal abortion is always classified as having an avoidable factor attributed to the patient.

Cause of death

Taking into account each contributory cause of death identified by the regional and central assessors, a single main cause of death has been allotted and subsequently classified according to the *International Classification of Diseases, Injuries and Causes of Death* (ICD) (WHO, 1977, see Appendix A1). During the years under review the 8th revision of this classification was current and was accordingly used by the Registrar General in the routine statistical analyses of maternal causes of death as reported on death certificates.

On 1 January 1979 this was superseded by the 9th revision (ICD 9) which included a major reconstruction of the chapter (XI) relating to conditions of pregnancy, childbirth and the puerperium with the provision of considerably more detail. In view to the potential advantages it was decided to use the ninth revision, in preference of the eighth, in the preparation of the data for this report although it was not in general use at the time. For comparative purposes the appropriate death certificates were re-coded to the ninth revision and an analysis of them is also included in Appendix A1 of this report. Since more information is available to the assessors the main cause of death allocated by them is not necessarily the same as the underlying cause shown on the death certficate which is the basis of the analysis by the Registrar General. Thus, one important change in this report affects deaths specifically attributable to 'complications of the administration of anaesthetic or other sedation in labour and delivery'. These are now allocated to a new category (ICD 668) whereas they were previously classified to the condition necessitating the procedure for which the anaesthetic was given. For the purposes of this enquiry this category has also been taken to include anaesthetic deaths associated with ectopic pregnancy or abortion.

6

The classification of maternal deaths

There is now international agreement to sub-divide obstetric deaths into direct and indirect. ICD 9 defines *direct* obstetric deaths as 'those resulting from obstetric complications of the pregnant state (pregnancy, labour and puerperium), from interventions, omissions, incorrect treatment, or from a chain of events resulting from any of the above'. *Indirect* obstetric deaths are defined as 'those resulting from previous existing disease, or disease that developed during pregnancy and which was not due to direct obstetric causes, but which was aggravated by physiologic effects of pregnancy'. Only those deaths from other causes which fortuitously occur in pregnancy or the puerperium are excluded from maternal mortality as internationally defined.

The present international definition of *direct* obstetric deaths almost equates with that of *true* maternal deaths as used previously; thus in this report the two terms are used interchangeably. The classification of *associated* maternal deaths in previous reports included other cases where the deceased was known to have been pregnant at the time of death or had been pregnant within one year of death. This is now sub-divided into two parts. Those cases where the existing disease and the pregnancy or puerperium were inter-related are defined as *indirect* obstetric deaths, the remainder are defined as *fortuitous* deaths. The new classification has helped to overcome some of the difficulties noted in the previous reports in which a death was classified as associated even if the pregnancy had brought to light or exacerbated the condition. These deaths now form an important part of the group of indirect obstetric deaths. There were 6 deaths which the assessors considered met the criteria for indirect (and hence associated) deaths but for which the most suitable ICD code was a direct obstetric cause.

For many of the deaths it is evident that several causes, in addition to the main cause of death, acted together. Each death where a particular cause contributed, directly or indirectly, is discussed in the chapter dealing with that cause, and may appear in the tables of more than one chapter. For example, a death where a hypertensive disease of pregnancy, haemorrhage and anaesthesia have all played a part would be counted in the tables in each of these chapters although the main cause of death would be hypertensive disease.

A further recommendation of ICD 9 defines a maternal death as 'the death of a woman while pregnant or within 42 days of termination of pregnancy, irrespective of the duration and the site of the pregnancy, from any cause related to or aggravated by the pregnancy or its management but not from accidental or incidental causes'. This is in line with the definition adopted by the International Federation of Gynaecology and Obstetrics (FIGO) and included in previous reports. In the Confidential Enquiry a maternal death has always been defined as 'one occurring during pregnancy or during labour or as a consequence of pregnancy within one year of delivery or abortion'. This wider definition has the advantage of including deaths in which the period of survival was longer than 42 days but in which the pregnancy had played an important role. However it does include deaths several months after delivery which are totally unconnected with the pregnancy. There are 75 cases included in the enquiry which do not meet the time constraints of these international definitions (see Table 1.7). These cases are also specifically identified in each chapter of this report.

Death rates

Statistics of the number of births are readily available from civil registration and are published annually by the Registrar General. The number of births is not however the best available denominator for women at risk of dying during pregnancy or childbirth, and in this report deaths are usually related to the number of *maternities*. Maternities are a count of the number of mothers who delivered as distinct from the number of babies born, and hence corrects for twins and other multiple births. The recent trends in maternities by age and parity (Figures IB, IC and ID) clearly follow those for births.

The provision in the tables of successive reports of death rates per million maternities has facilitated appropriate comparisons with reports from earlier triennia during which birth rates were higher. This practice has been continued in this report in tables where the number of deaths is sufficient to give meaningful rates, but small numbers have precluded its use in those tables sub-divided into age or parity. For these an alternative technique has been adopted whereby data are given for the number of *expected deaths* on the basis of age (or parity)—specific death rates for a total number of earlier years (usually the period 1967 – 1975). This allows direct comparison with the *number of actual deaths* in the current triennium. It also facilitates the computation of the over-all effect of age or parity on the death rates for the various causes of death making use of extended series of data over a period of 12 years (for example see Table 2.2 and 2.3).

For deaths associated with abortion and ectopic pregnancy (Table 11.2) an alternative denominator has been used which reflects the estimated number of conceptions rather than the total number of births. This has been calculated by adding the numbers of maternities and legal terminations to those of ectopic pregnancies and spontaneous abortions admitted to NHS hospitals (DHSS, OPCS, Welsh Office, 1981).

Parity

As in previous reports, parity is defined as the number of previous preg-nancies of 28 weeks gestation or more (regardless of the outcome of the preg-nancy) plus the present pregnancy, whatever its duration. Thus, a woman with one previous stillbirth and one live child who dies from an ectopic pregnancy at 12 weeks gestation is defined as para 3; whereas another woman who dies in her fourth pregnancy after three previous abortions would be regarded as para 1. It is necessary to define parity in this way as no information about the numbers of previous abortions and ectopic pregnancies is collected at birth registration in England and Wales the statistics which form the basis of the denominators in this report.

8

Figure 1B *Number of maternities by age-group 1961-1978*

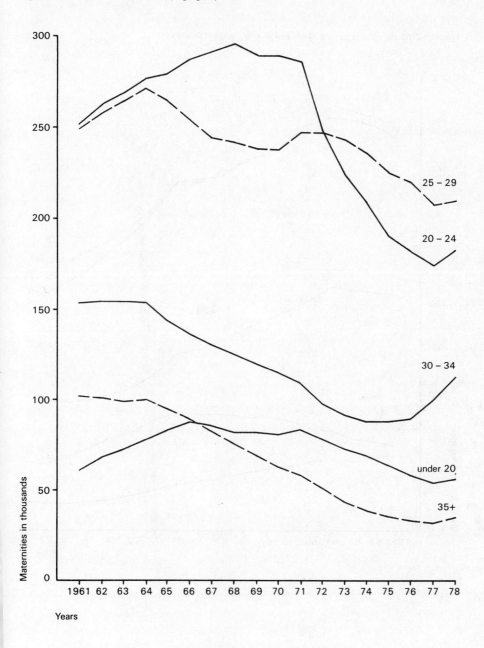

9

Figure 1C *Maternity rate per 1000 women in age-groups 1961-1978*

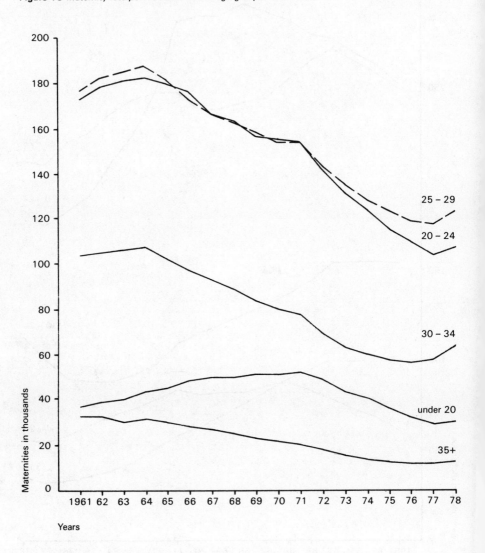

Figure 1D *Number of maternities according to parity 1963-1978*

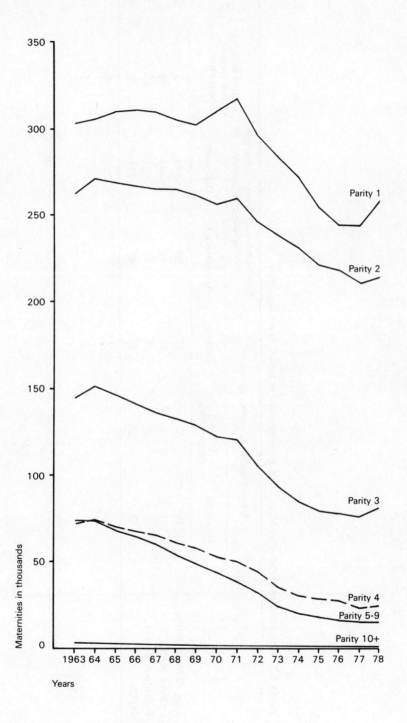

Table 1.7: *Reported deaths in relation to stage of pregnancy at which death occurred*

	Deaths under 28 weeks gestation			Deaths from 28 weeks gestation to 6 weeks postpartum		Deaths later than 6 weeks postpartum	Total
	Abortions	Ectopic pregnancies	Others	Undelivered	Delivered		
True (Direct) deaths	19	22	15	22	140	9	227
Indirect deaths	11	0	12	11	44	19	97
Fortuitous deaths	2	0	13	14	27	47	103
TOTAL	32	22	40	47	211	75	427

Furthermore, information about previous births is confined to the registration of legitimate births. Thus the construction of a parity distribution of all maternities (Appendices A4 and A7) requires the allocation of illegitimate births by parity. This is done on the assumption that for mothers under 16 years of age it is the first birth, and that for older women the parity distribution is the same as for legitimate births at a similar age.

The 1976 – 78 series

The 427 deaths on which sufficient information was available were classified as:—

227 (53 per cent) true (or direct) deaths;
97 (23 ,, ,,) indirect deaths; and
103 (24 ,, ,,) fortuitous deaths.

Table 1.7 shows that about one death in eight (12 per cent) was associated with abortion or ectopic pregnancy, and a further ten per cent of deaths were of women who died undelivered before the 28th week of pregnancy. In all 141 (33 per cent) died before delivery of a potentially viable child.

In the triennium the number of deaths which occurred more than six weeks after delivery was greater than in 1973 – 75. More than half of these (63 per cent) were fortuitous deaths which have probably been more assiduously reported than on previous occasions.

Table 1.8 shows that the maternal mortality rate associated with true deaths varies quite considerably between Regions—from 18 per 100,000 births in North East Thames, which has now remained at this level for two triennia, to 5.4 per 100,000 in Wessex.

Table 1.8: *Reported true deaths, total births and true maternal mortality rate 1976 – 78 (deaths from abortion and anaesthesia associated with abortion in parentheses)*

Regional Health Authority	Reportedϕ true deaths		Total births	True maternal† mortality rate	Reported indirect
Northern	19	(2)	112,224	15.1	9
Yorkshire	16	(–)	128,915	12.4	8
Trent	19	(–)	161,946	11.7	6
East Anglian	11	(1)	66,059	15.1	3
North West Thames	16	(1)	128,531	11.7	6
North East Thames	30	(5)	138,523	18.0	2
South East Thames	11	(1)	123,782	8.1	3
South West Thames	15	(1)	94,945	14.7	6
Wessex	5	(–)	92,097	5.4	2
Oxford	10	(–)	87,084	11.5	4
South Western	10	(–)	105,389	9.5	6
West Midlands	25	(4)	189,452	11.1	15
Mersey	11	(1)	89,028	11.2	3
North Western	21	(2)	147,167	12.9	10
Wales	7	(1)	99,432	6.0	14
England and Wales	227	(19)	1,766,169	11.9	97

ϕ Only one additional death known to the Registrar General was not reported.

† Excluding abortions and anaesthetic deaths associated with abortions, per 100,000 total births.

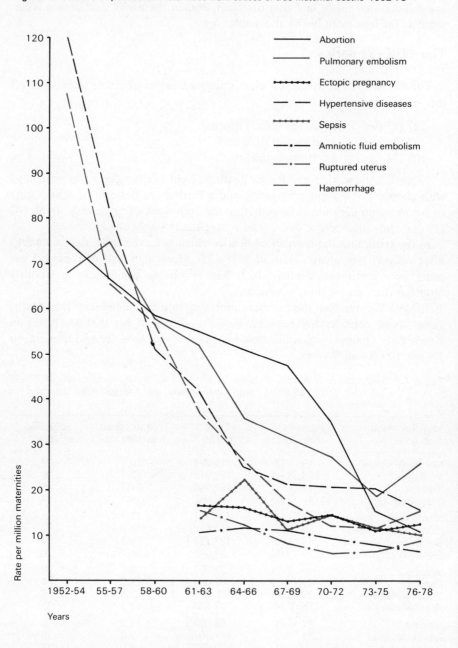

Figure 1E *Death rates per million maternities from causes of true maternal deaths 1952-78*

Legend:
- Abortion
- Pulmonary embolism
- Ectopic pregnancy
- Hypertensive diseases
- Sepsis
- Amniotic fluid embolism
- Ruptured uterus
- Haemorrhage

Y-axis: Rate per million maternities

X-axis: Years — 1952-54, 55-57, 58-60, 61-63, 64-66, 67-69, 70-72, 73-75, 76-78

Table 1.9: *Main causes of true maternal deaths (i.e. directly due to pregnancy or childbirth), 1952 – 78*

Causes	1952 – 54	1955 – 57	1958 – 60	1961 – 63	1964 – 66	1967 – 69	1970 – 72	1973 – 75	1976 – 78	Excluded under International* definition 1976 – 78
	Numbers of deaths (Rates per million maternities in parentheses)									
Abortion	153 (74.5)	141 (66.7)	135 (58.8)	139 (55.1)	133 (51.1)	117 (47.6)	81 (35.2)	29 (15.1)	19‡ (10.9)	1
Pulmonary embolism	138 (67.2)	157 (74.3)	132 (57.5)	129 (51.2)	91 (35.0)	75 (30.5)	61 (26.5)	35 (18.2)	45 (25.7)	2
Haemorrhage	220† (107.2)†	138 (65.3)	130 (56.7)	92 (36.5)	68 (26.2)	41 (16.7)	27 (11.7)	21 (10.9)	26 (14.9)	1
Hypertensive diseases of pregnancy	246 (119.8)	171 (80.9)	118 (51.4)	104 (41.3)	67 (25.8)	53 (21.6)	47 (20.5)	39 (20.3)	29 (16.6)	–
All other causes	369 (179.7)	254 (120.2)	227 (98.9)	228 (90.5)	220 (84.6)	169 (68.8)	139 (60.5)	111 (57.8)	108 (61.7)	5
Total	1,094 (532.9)	861 (407.4)	742 (323.4)	692 (274.6)	579 (222.7)	455 (185.2)	355 (154.5)	235 (122.3)	227 (129.8)	9

* See page 7
† corrected figures
‡ Including 5 deaths from anaesthesia associated with operations for abortion for comparison with previous triennia

15

Table 1.10: *True maternal deaths from other than main causes, 1961 – 78*

Causes	1961 – 63	1964 – 66	1967 – 69	1970 – 72	1973 – 75	1976 – 78	Excluded under International* definition 1976 – 78
	Numbers of deaths (Rates per million maternities in parentheses)						
Ectopic pregnancy	42 (16.7)	42 (16.2)	32 (13.0)	34 (14.8)	20 (10.4)	22‡ (12.6)	–
Sepsis (excluding abortion with sepsis)	33 (13.1)	57 (21.9)	26 (10.6)	32 (13.9)	22 (11.4)	17 (9.7)	2
Amniotic fluid embolism	27 (10.7)	30 (11.5)	27 (11.0)	22 (9.6)	14 (7.3)	11 (6.3)	–
Ruptured uterus	38 (15.1)	30 (11.5)	18 (7.3)	12 (5.2)	11 (5.7)	14 (8.0)	–
Miscellaneous causes	88 (34.9)	61 (23.5)	66 (26.9)	39 (17.0)	44 (22.9)	20 (11.4)	1
Deaths associated with anaesthesia (excluding operations for abortion and ectopic pregnancy)						24 (13.7)	2
Total	228 (90.5)	220 (84.6)	169 (68.8)	139 (60.5)	111 (57.8)	108 (61.8)	5

* See page 7

‡ Including one death from anaesthesia associated with operations for ectopic pregnancy for comparison with previous triennia

Figure 1E shows the death rates per million maternities for the main causes of true maternal death, with Table 1.9 giving four causes which have been the most important since 1952. Abortion has been included to provide continuity with the previous triennia, although between 1976–78 there were only 14 deaths directly attributed to abortion, with a further 5 deaths from anaesthesia associated with operations for abortion. Pulmonary embolism was the most frequent cause of death in this triennium, and there was an increase in the mortality rate from 18.2 per million maternities in 1973–75 to 25.7 in 1976–78. There was also an increase in the death rate from haemorrhage from 10.9 in 1973–75 to 14.9 in 1976–78.

Table 1.10 shows the other causes of true maternal death. For the first time in 1976–78, deaths directly associated with anaesthesia have been separately classified and coded and have not been included with the miscellaneous deaths under the indications for operations. There was a small decline in numbers and rates of death from sepsis and amniotic fluid embolism, and a small rise in deaths from ruptured uterus.

These clinical findings are discussed in the succeeding chapters and summarized in Chapter 17.

References

Department of Health and Social Security, 1979.
  Report on confidential enquiries into maternal deaths in England and Wales 1973 – 75 (Report on Health and Social Subjects No 14) London, HMSO.
Department of Health and Social Security, Office of Population Censuses and Surveys, Welsh Office, 1981.
  Hospital In-patient Enquiry 1978. Series MB4 No 12, London, HMSO.
Office of Population Censuses and Surveys, 1980a.
  Birth Statistics 1978 FM1 No 5. London, HMSO.
Office of Population Censuses and Surveys, 1980b.
  Mortality Statistics: Childhood and Maternity 1978. London, HMSO.
Office of Population Censuses and Surveys, 1980c.
  Abortion Statistics 1978 Series AB No 5. London, HMSO.
World Health Organization, 1977.
  Manual of the International Statistical Classification of diseases, injuries and causes of death (9th revision)
  Geneva, World Health Organization.

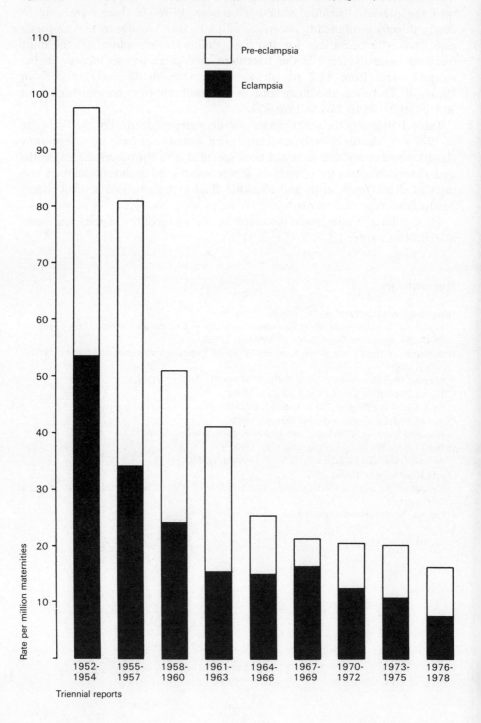

Figure 2 *Death rate per million maternities from hypertensive diseases of pregnancy 1952-1978*

2. Hypertensive diseases of pregnancy*

Pre-eclampsia and eclampsia

During the years 1976 – 78 there were 29 deaths from pre-eclampsia and eclampsia (ICD 642). This compares with 39 such deaths in 1973 – 75 and 47 during 1970 – 72. There were 13 deaths associated with eclamptic fits during 1976 – 78 compared with 21 in 1973 – 75 and 29 in 1970 – 72. (Table 2.1)

Table 2.1: *Number of women who died from hypertensive diseases of pregnancy and the death rate per million maternities, 1952 – 1978.*

Triennium	Total		Pre-eclampsia		Eclampsia	
	No	Rate	No	Rate	No	Rate
1952 – 54	200	97.4	90	43.8	110	53.6
1955 – 57	171	80.9	99	46.8	72	34.1
1958 – 60	118	51.4	63	27.0	56	24.4
1961 – 63	104	41.3	64	25.4	40	15.9
1964 – 66	67	25.8	27	10.4	40	15.4
1967 – 69	53	21.6	12	4.9	41	16.7
1970 – 72	47	20.5	18	7.8	29	12.6
1973 – 75	39	20.3	18	9.4	21	10.9
1976 – 78	29	16.6	16	9.1	13	7.4

It is noteworthy that the death rate per million maternities continued to fall for deaths from all hypertensive diseases of pregnancy, as shown in Figure 2.

Hypertensive diseases of pregnancy occurred in 15 cases in which death was directly attributable to another cause. These have been excluded from this chapter and are included in the following chapters:—

Haemorrhage	5
Amniotic fluid embolism	2
Pulmonary embolism	2
Anaesthesia	2
Ruptured uterus	1
Cardiac disease associated with pregnancy	1
Deaths from associated causes { Phaeochromocytoma / Diabetes Mellitus	2

*Prior to the 1973 – 1975 report this chapter has been entitled 'Toxaemia of Pregnancy (Pre-eclampsia and eclampsia)'.

There were also two patients with essential hypertension. The main cause of death in both cases was haemorrhage and they have been included in Chapter 3.

Deaths assigned to hypertensive diseases of pregnancy may be due to a direct complication of the condition or to a complication of management, such as Caesarean section, made necessary by the disease.

Duration of pregnancy

Three women died *undelivered*. One died at home of asphyxia in eclampsia at the 34th week of pregnancy. She had concealed the pregnancy and was attending her general practitioner for excessive weight gain and oedema. Two women died of cerebral haemorrhage following pre-eclampsia, the hypertension occurring in both at the 26th week of gestation. One of these 2 patients had no antenatal care and died 2 hours after going to the emergency department of a hospital. The other died while being treated as an in-patient in a consultant obstetric unit at the 30th week.

The duration of pregnancy in weeks at the time of delivery in the remaining 26 patients who were delivered was:

Duration of pregnancy in weeks at time of delivery	Number of women who died after delivery	
	Pre-eclampsia	Eclampsia
27 – 28	1	1
29 – 30	1	3
31 – 32	1	1
33 – 34	3	2
35 – 36	2	1
37 – 38	4	–
39 – 40	2	3
41 – 42	–	1
Total	14	12

Fetal loss

Of the 26 patients who were delivered, 10 babies were stillborn, 16 were born alive but there were 2 neonatal deaths, one at 30 minutes and one at 12 hours after delivery. The perinatal mortality was 46.2%, similar to 46.5% for 1973 – 75, as compared with 37.8% for the triennium 1970 – 72.

Actual cause of death

During 1976 – 78 there were 13 deaths in which fits occurred and in all cases but one a postmortem examination was performed. In this one instance permission was refused. In the remaining 12, the mortality was caused by a complication directly associated with the condition as follows:—

Cerebral haemorrhage	8 cases
Cerebral oedema	2 cases
Asphyxia	1 case
Anoxic cardiac arrest	1 case

There were 16 deaths due to pre-eclampsia all being directly attributable to recognized complications of hypertensive diseases of pregnancy as follows:—

Cerebral haemorrhage	9 cases
Anoxic cardiac arrest	2 cases
Hepato-renal failure	1 case
Adrenal cortical haemorrhage	1 case
Disseminated intravascular coagulation	1 case
Cerebral infarction	1 case
Cerebellar infarction and pituitary necrosis	1 case

The management of hypertensive diseases of pregnancy may be responsible for a train of events which ends in death from causes other than those listed above. For example, prolonged bed rest followed by operative delivery may result in venous thrombosis and death from pulmonary embolism. Twenty one (72%) of the deaths were ascribed to cerebral pathology, of which 17 were caused by cerebral haemorrhage. Thus haemorrhagic stroke is by far the most important factor leading to death. This continues the pattern which has been demonstrated in previous Enquiries, and cerebral haemorrhage is a well defined complication of extreme hypertension. This pattern of maternal mortality underlines the importance of controlling maternal hypertension by medical means even in the relatively short interval between diagnosis and delivery.

Several operative deliveries had to be undertaken quickly. Twelve of the 26 women had a Caesarean section, 4 had a forceps delivery and one a vacuum (ventouse) extraction. There was no multiple pregnancy.

Age and parity

For 1967 – 78 the death rate per million maternities from hypertensive disease of pregnancy for women over 35 years of age was 43.8 compared with 18.1 for women under 35. Also for 1967 – 78 the death rate per million maternities from primigravidae was 31.5 compared with 12.0 for women having their second or subsequent babies.

Tables 2.2 and 2.3 show that within the overall fall in death rate, there were some minor differences between the present distribution of age and parity compared with earlier years as reflected in the 'expected' deaths. None of these are, however, statistically significant.

Table 2.2: *Number of women who died from hypertensive diseases of pregnancy by age, 1976 – 78, compared with 1967 – 75*

	1967 – 1975			1976 – 1978		
Age (Years)	Total maternities	Number of deaths	Rate per million	†Expected deaths on basis of 1967 – 75 rates	Total maternities	Number of actual deaths
25	3,030,081	54	17.8	36	709,038	11
25 – 29	2,161,981	36	16.7	11	637,683	15
30 – 34	967,641	23	23.8	7	303,575	2
35 – 39	402,193	22	54.7	1	79,622	–
40 +	115,315	4	34.7	1	18,931	1
All ages	6,677,211	139		Total (by Addition) 36	1,748,849	29

Table 2.3: *Number of women who died from hypertensive diseases of pregnancy by parity* 1976 – 78, compared with 1967 – 75*

	1967 – 1975			1976 – 1978		
Parity	Total maternities	Number of deaths	Rate per million	†Expected deaths on basis of 1967 – 75 rates	Total maternities	Number of actual deaths
1	2,680,166	88	32.8	25	747,409	20
2	2,230,024	17	7.6	5	643,922	5
3	998,707	14	14.0	3	233,388	2
4	417,750	8	19.2	1	76,247	–
5 +	350,564	12	34.2	2	47,885	2
All	6,677,211	139		Total (by Addition) 36	1,748,849	29

* For definition of parity see page 8
† For explanation of method of calculation see page 8

Frequency of fits

Thirteen women were recorded as having had fits. With one exception all of the fits were witnessed by professional observers. One woman had fits at home during a concealed pregnancy and died from asphyxia. In 7 women fits occurred only during pregnancy, during labour in one woman, and postnatally in 2 women. In 3 other women fits occurred both in pregnancy and post-natally.

Number of fits before death	Number of women
1	4
2	5
3	1
4	1
5	1
'Many'	1

Racial characteristics

Three of the patients who died were born abroad. One was born in India and one in Pakistan and they had had virtually no antenatal care. One woman from Tanzania had been in England for three months only, but then had attended hospital fairly regularly. A fourth patient born in the United Kingdom, but of West Indian parentage had received almost no antenatal care.

Avoidable factors

One or more avoidable factors were considered to be present in 21 (72%) of the 29 deaths directly caused by hypertensive diseases of pregnancy. Of the 21 women 13 had eclampsia and the remaining 8 had pre-eclampsia.

Percentage of cases with avoidable factors 1952 – 78

1952 – 55	52%	1967 – 69	66%
1953 – 57	55%	1970 – 72	66%
1958 – 60	56%	1973 – 75	74%
1961 – 63	49%	1976 – 78	72%
1964 – 66	56%		

The presence of one or more avoidable factors in 72% of all deaths directly caused by hypertensive diseases of pregnancy indicates that the standard of care fell short of that which is generally accepted as being satisfactory.

In the 13 fatalities in which eclampsia occurred, one or more avoidable factors were present in each case and the responsibility was distributed as follows:—

The patient alone was involved 3 times.
The patient and general practitioner were involved in one.
The patient and consultant were involved in one.
The general practitioner alone was involved twice.
The general practitioner and consultant were involved in 3.
The consultant alone was involved twice.
The consultant and anaesthetist were involved in one.

Thus the patient was involved in 5 instances, the general practitioner in 6, the consultant in 6 and the anaesthetist in one. In no case was a midwife involved.

In each instance when an avoidable factor was attributed to the patient either she was at fault in concealing the pregnancy, having no antenatal care, failed to attend when advised or neglected instructions.

An avoidable factor was attributed to the general practitioner when the patient was only seen in an irregular haphazard fashion despite warning signs of hypertensive diseases of pregnancy. There was failure to seek the opinion of a consultant and delay in admitting the patient to a consultant unit for careful observation and management. These factors resulted in the death from eclampsia of 5 primigravidae booked for delivery in separate general practitioner units. A further comment concerning these women is in Chapter 16.

Consultant responsibility involves all the medical staff of an obstetric unit. Junior staff were at fault in not informing the consultant of one patient with fulminating pre-eclampsia. In one case the consultant in charge did not see the patient either at her antenatal visits, or when she was admitted to his unit at the 36th week of pregnancy with blood pressure of 200/130 mm Hg and proteinuria. This lack of concern continued during the 2 weeks before she had a Caesarean section at the 38th week of pregnancy by a senior Registrar. In another case the consultant agreed to share with a general practitioner the care of a woman who had had pre-eclampsia at the 32nd week of a previous pregnancy. Her blood pressure in the fatal pregnancy was 150/100 mm Hg at the 14th week of gestation and 230/120 mm Hg at the 28th week. She died of cerebral haemorrhage at the 29th week after a Caesarean section by a registrar.

In patients with hypertensive diseases of pregnancy without fits there were 8 instances of one or more avoidable factors as follows:

The patient alone was involved twice.
The consultant alone was involved 4 times.
The consultant and general practitioner were involved twice.
There was no midwife concerned with any avoidable factor.

Phaeochromocytoma

One case occurred during 1976 – 78 and as in previous reports is mentioned here. In this case the raised blood pressure 160/100 mm Hg simulated hypertensive disease of pregnancy and the disease was not recognized. This case is described in chapter 14.

Summary and conclusions

1. There were 29 deaths directly caused by hypertensive diseases of pregnancy during 1975 – 78 and this continues the progressive decline in the number of such deaths since 1952.

2. There was a greater fall in the number of women dying from eclampsia than in women dying from pre-eclampsia.

3. One or more avoidable factors were considered to be present in 72% of deaths directly caused by hypertensive diseases of pregnancy.

4. Cerebral haemorrhage is the commonest cause of death in the hypertensive diseases of pregnancy.

3. Haemorrhage

There were 26 deaths directly due to haemorrhage in the triennium 1976 – 78; these are included in the figures shown in Appendix A, Table A1, as follows:

ICD 641.0   Antepartum haemorrhage   { Abruptio placentae   6
                                          Placenta praevia }   2   8
ICD 666.0   Postpartum haemorrhage associated with retained placenta   1
ICD 666.1   Other immediate postpartum haemorrhage   13
ICD 666.2   Delayed and secondary postpartum   3
ICD 665   Delivery with other obstetrical trauma   1

Table 3.1 shows the number of deaths recorded in each of the triennial reports as directly caused by haemorrhage, with the corresponding death rate per million maternities.

Table 3.1: *Number of deaths from haemorrhage and rate per million maternities, 1952 – 1978*

	Triennial reports								
	1952 – 54	1955 – 57	1958 – 60	1961 – 63	1964 – 66	1967 – 69	1970 – 72	1973 – 75	1976 – 78
Placental abruption	78	40	44	25	27	16	6	6	6
Placenta praevia	29	28	25	23	16	9	6	2	2
Postpartum haemorrhage	113	70	61	44	25	16	15	13	18
Total	220	138	130	92	68	41	27	21	26
Rate per million maternities	107.2	65.3	59.7	36.5	26.2	16.7	11.7*	10.9	14.9

* *Note correction since last Report.*

The death rate from haemorrhage is shown in Figure 3. The number of deaths from haemorrhage and the death rate from haemorrhage have both increased since the last report. Although the number of deaths from placental abruption and placenta praevia has not changed, there has been an increase in the number of deaths from postpartum haemorrhage, the number at 18 being the highest since the 1964 – 66 triennium.

Figure 3 *Death rate per million maternities from haemorrhage 1952-1978*

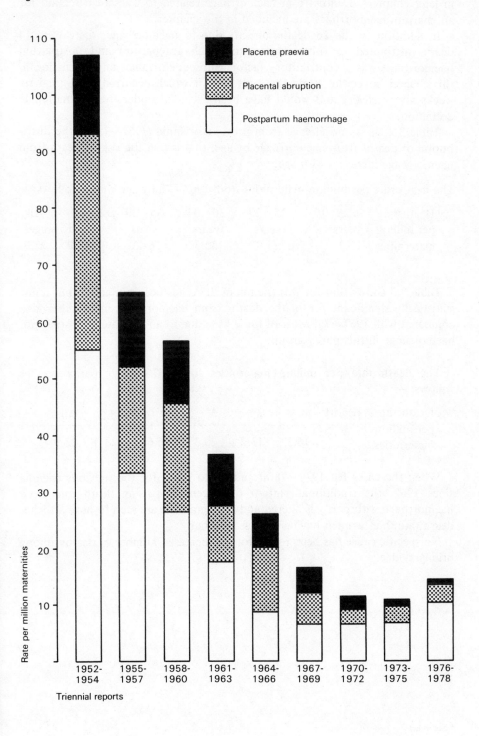

As in previous reports, deaths from haemorrhage attributed to abortion, ectopic pregnancy or ruptured uterus are not included here, but are discussed in later chapters. Deaths from haemorrhage related to Caesarean section for antepartum haemorrhage are included in this chapter.

In addition to the 26 deaths directly due to haemorrhage, there were 14 deaths attributed to other causes, to which antepartum and postpartum haemorrhage was a contributory factor. Subsequent tables and discussion in this chapter cover the 40 deaths, only one of which occurred more than six weeks after delivery and would have been excluded under the international* definition.

Table 3.2 shows no change from previous triennia (1967 – 75) in the distribution of deaths from haemorrhage by age; that is that the risk of death from haemorrhage increases with age.

The death rate per million maternities from 1967 – 78 by age was as follows:—

Death rate per million maternities	< 25 years	25 – 29 years	30 – 34 years	35 – 39 years	40 years	All ages
	12.3	18.9	32.3	64.3	163.9	22.9

Table 3.3 shows that for this triennium there has been a marked, but a not statistically significant rise in the deaths from haemorrhage in primigravidae compared with 1967 – 75. Most of these were due to an increase in postpartum haemorrhage in this parity group.

The death rate per million maternities for 1967 – 78 by parity was as follows:—

Death rate per million maternities	Parity 1	2	3	4	5 +	All
	16.3	13.2	20.3	46.6	128.0	22.9

When the cases for 1976 – 78 are added to those for the previous triennia since 1967, the traditional pattern of a generally rising death rate from haemorrhage with parity is altered and primigravidae are seen to have a higher death rate than women having their second baby.

No specific cause has been found for the increased number of deaths among primigravidae.

* See page 7

Table 3.2: *Number of women who died from haemorrhage by age 1976 – 78 compared with 1967 – 75*

Age	1967 – 1975				Total mater-nities	Number of actual deaths	1976 – 1978		
	Total mater-nities	Number of deaths	Rate per million	†Expected deaths on basis of 1967 – 75 rates			Placental abruption	Placenta praevia	Post-partum haemorrage
<25	3,030,081	35	11.6	8	709,038	11	1	–	10
25 – 29	2,161,981	39	18.0	11	637,683	14	1	3	10
30 – 34	967,641	32	33.1	10	303,575	9	4	1	4
35 – 39	402,193	27	67.1	5	79,622	4	–	1	3
40 +	115,315	20	173.4	3	18,931	2	2	1	–
All ages	6,677,211	153		Total (by addition) 37	1,748,849	40	8	5	27

† For explanation of method of calculation see page 8

29

Table 3.3: *Number of women who died from haemorrhage by parity 1976–78 compared with 1967–75*

Parity	1967 – 1975				1976 – 78				
	Total maternities	Number of deaths	Rate per million	†Expected deaths on basis of 1967–75 rates	Total maternities	Total number of actual deaths	Placental abruption	Placenta praevia	Post-partum haemorrhage
1	2,680,166	32	11.9	9	747,409	24	3	1	20
2	2,230,024	34	15.2	10	643,922	4	1	1	2
3	998,707	22	22.0	5	233,388	3	–	1	2
4	417,750	22	52.7	4	76,247	1	–	1	–
5+	350,564	43	122.7	6	47,885	8	4	1	3
Not stated	–	–	–	–	–	–	–	–	–
All	6,677,211	153	–	Total (by addition) 34	1,748,849	40	8	5	27

† For explanation of method of calculation see page 8

Table 3.4 shows the frequency of deaths with avoidable factors from each cause, the overall percentage with avoidable factors 65% being a slight reduction from 71% for 1973 – 75.

Table 3.4: *Deaths associated with haemorrhage—frequency of avoidable* factors*

	Total deaths	Number of deaths with avoidable factors	Frequency (%)
Placental abruption	8	5	63
Placenta praevia	5	2	40
Postpartum haemorrhage	27	19	70
Total	40	26	65

Placental abruption

There were 6 deaths caused by placental abruption and in addition, placental abruption occurred in 2 other deaths, one due to amniotic fluid embolism and the other associated with anaesthesia.

There were no avoidable factors in two of the six deaths primarily due to placental abruption. One of these two patients collapsed at home at the 37th week of her first pregnancy. She seemed dead but was resuscitated by mouth-to-mouth breathing and external cardiac massage. When admitted to hospital her abdomen seemed excessively distended and she was delivered of a stillborn infant by classical Caesarean section. Some retroplacental clot was found and there was free blood and gas in the abdomen. A coagulation defect developed and the patient died soon afterwards. Amniotic fluid embolism was suspected but not confirmed histologically. The other patient was well until she suddenly developed severe headache at 36 weeks and was comatose when admitted to a maternity hospital where intracranial haemorrhage was diagnosed. She was transferred to the neurosurgical unit in another city but died soon after admission. Autopsy revealed widespread bleeding, including multiple cerebral haemorrhages, bleeding into the liver and lungs and a large concealed placental abruption which had predisposed to the disseminated intravascular clotting which caused the other haemorrhages.

Of the 8 patients who died with placental abruption, 3 died undelivered, one was delivered spontaneously, one by forceps and 3 by Caesarean section. Five of these patients developed a coagulation disorder.

Avoidable factors were present in 5 cases.

In two instances the patient was considered to be involved. One refused admission to hospital at the 26th week of pregnancy although her blood

* See Chapter 1

pressure was 190/120 mm Hg; she subsequently suffered severe placental abruption and was dead on admission. The other patient failed to attend the antenatal clinic until vaginal bleeding began at the 24th week of her 11th pregnancy. Three of her previous 5 pregnancies had been complicated by placental abruption. Later, when signs of severe placental abruption developed, Caesarean section was performed. An avoidable factor was attributed to the consultant team because of delay with blood transfusion at operation, blood being withheld because of the patient's hypertension.

The consultant obstetric team was involved in 2 other cases. In one, junior obstetric staff failed to recognize placental abruption in a patient being treated for suspected premature labour. Although the consultant recognized that the patient was in shock this proved irreversible and the patient died despite extensive blood transfusion and hysterectomy. In the other case involving a consultant team, avoidable factors were attributed to delayed and inadequate resuscitation of a patient with severe placental abruption and delay in proceeding with operative delivery.

The anaesthetist was considered to be involved in a case described in Chapter 8 when an anaesthetic was given for Caesarean section because of acute fetal distress associated with placental abruption.

Placenta praevia

There were 2 deaths from haemorrhage due to placenta praevia and 3 deaths from other causes in which placenta praevia was an important factor. One patient was admitted to hospital at 30 weeks gestation with antepartum haemorrhage. Two of her four previous deliveries had been by Caesarean section. Vaginal bleeding continued and she was again delivered by Caesarean section when an anterior placenta praevia was found. Bleeding was profuse but haemostasis seemed to be satisfactory at the end of the operation. Blood loss continued after operation and despite blood replacement and oxytocin infusion cardiac arrest occurred and was corrected. A uterine pack was inserted and did not control the bleeding. After sub-total hysterectomy the patient died from a second cardiac arrest.

Another woman who had had 3 previous Caesarean sections for disproportion had an elective classical Caesarean section for a confirmed placenta praevia. The operation was performed by a registrar. There was profuse and uncontrollable bleeding when the placenta was removed; it appeared unusually adherent to the previous lower segment scars. Packing the lower segment and uterus did not control bleeding. A senior registrar and consultant were called and commenced hysterectomy. Operation was difficult because the bladder was adherent to the previous scars. Bleeding could not be controlled and despite infusion of 17 units of blood the patient died.

A woman, aged 27, was delivered by elective Caesarean section at term in her third pregnancy, because of placenta praevia and breech presentation. Operation was uneventful, but anaesthetic factors led to the patient's lungs being over-inflated at the end of the procedure and she died of a gas embolism. The case is included in Chapter 8.

Another patient who had a cervical suture inserted in early pregnancy was delivered by emergency lower segment Caesarean section because of severe antepartum haemorrhage. Following delivery, the patient developed pyrexia. Her condition rapidly deteriorated, with rigors and septic shock. Despite intensive, appropriate treatment she died 9 days after delivery. Autopsy confirmed the presence of septicaemia, the organisms being anaerobic streptococci and bacteroides. The case is included in Chapter 12.

The fifth patient suffered from Eisenmenger's defect, and her pregnancy was managed in hospital from the 28th week, cardiac failure being treated by digoxin, diuretics and repeated small venesections. Pulmonary embolism was suspected at 33 weeks. Severe antepartum haemorrhage occurred soon afterwards in association with preterm labour. This was deliberately allowed to progress for 4 hours in the hope that Caesarean section could be avoided, but continued bleeding made operative delivery essential. At delivery placenta praevia was confirmed, and there was a further blood loss of 2 litres. Ten units of blood and 4 units of plasma were infused but the patient died from cardiac and respiratory arrest. The case is included in Chapter 6.

Avoidable factors were considered to be present in two cases. In one patient having her fourth Caesarean section and known to have a placenta praevia, it would have been appropriate for the procedure to have been performed, or supervised by the consultant. In the other case, avoidable factors were considered to involve the anaesthetic management.

Postpartum haemorrhage

There were 18 deaths directly caused by postpartum haemorrhage. In another 9 deaths postpartum haemorrhage contributed to the fatal outcome; 8 of these were true obstetric deaths and one an indirect death and they have been coded as follows:

ICD 642.5	Hypertensive diseases of pregnancy (severe pre-eclampsia)	3 cases
ICD 673.1	Amniotic fluid embolism	3 cases
ICD 668	Complications of the administration of anaesthetic in labour and delivery	2 cases
ICD 648.9 } 965.1 } E950.0 }	Other complications of pregnancy (self administered overdose)	1 case

A blood coagulation disorder was demonstrated in 12 of the 27 cases in which postpartum haemorrhage caused, or played a part in causing death. The coagulation disorder was usually associated with disseminated intravascular coagulation and defibrination. On one occasion, bleeding was made worse by heparin administration given for several days to correct suspected fibrinolysis. In another case, the coagulation disorder was associated with self poisoning by aspirin.

33

Amniotic fluid embolism was suspected in 6 cases, but only proved on histological examination of the lungs in 3 cases, described in Chapter 10. In one, a clinical picture of collapse, cyanosis, haemorrhage and coagulation disorder, proved to be caused by septicaemia.

Torrential haemorrhage was a feature in one death in which inversion of the uterus occurred. The umbilical cord broke while the midwife was attempting to deliver the placenta by controlled cord traction. When the placenta was expelled by fundal pressure it was found to be attached to the inverted fundus. The registrar could not correct the inversion at once and cardiac arrest occurred in the operating theatre before anaesthesia was commenced. Although the heart beat was started again and the inversion replaced under anaesthesia, the patient suffered brain damage and died within 4 hours. This case was coded to ICD 665.

Of the 27 women who died of postpartum haemorrhage, 7 were delivered spontaneously, 10 by forceps, one by vacuum extractor and 9 by Caesarean section, of which one was of 'classical' type. There were 3 sets of twins, and of the 30 children, 22 were born alive. There was one early neonatal death, one infant died at 6 weeks of age and there were 8 stillbirths.

The possibility was considered that the increased number of deaths from postpartum haemorrhage in this triennium might have been due to the discontinuance of a syntocinon infusion, if used, too soon after delivery. In 9 of the 17 deaths directly attributed to postpartum haemorrhage, Syntocinon had been infused intravenously, in 8 to induce and in one to augment labour. In 5 of the 9 women treated with intravenous Syntocinon there was no report of the infusion being continued after delivery of the infant, but in 3 of these 5 women, ergometrine, Syntocinon, or a combination of both had been administered by intravenous or intramuscular injection, in accord with accepted practice at delivery. Failure to administer oxytocin drugs appropriately did not therefore appear to be the cause of the excess of 'actual' compared with 'expected' deaths in 1976–78 (Tables 3.2 and 3.3).

Avoidable factors were considered to have been present in 19 deaths, in 7 of which there was more than one factor. Two patients were at fault. One grande multipara who suffered from cor pulmonale as well as agarophobia and depression, decided to manage her 7th pregnancy and delivery with the help of her husband and made no arrangements for medical or nursing care. An ambulance was called when a pre-term infant was delivered, but the patient refused admission. Later, a police surgeon was called and sent the patient into hospital by ambulance. She was moribund on admission, as a result of profuse haemorrhage and she died 2 hours after delivery. The infant also died. The other patient involved also died as a result of severe bleeding, following Caesarean section for multiple pregnancy. Blood transfusion was withheld at first because of the patient's religious convictions and this delay was considered an avoidable factor and attributed to the patient. Although she later agreed to the transfusion, the delay had endangered her life. The consultant team was also considered involved because the blood loss at operation was underestimated.

General practitioners were involved in 2 cases in which patients were considered to have been wrongly booked for delivery in general practitioner units.

In one, the consultant team was also considered to be involved for accepting a booking for the GP unit. There were clear indications in pregnancy that labour might be difficult, because the patient was of short stature and the fetal head failed to engage. Operative delivery proved necessary and death was related to anaesthetic factors. In the other case the general practitioner was considered at fault for booking for a general practitioner delivery a patient in her 5th pregnancy, 6 years since her last confinement. During pregnancy she gained 19 Kg in weight and when hypertension and proteinuria developed at 38 weeks, she was only advised to rest at home. Placental abruption occurred and led to a sequence of events which finally culminated in her death from complications of postpartum haemorrhage.

Avoidable factors involved the anaesthetist in 5 cases which are considered in Chapter 8, although death was considered directly due to anaesthesia in only 2 of these cases.

The consultant team was involved in 16 cases, including the three already mentioned and involving general practitioners in two and the patient in one. In another case the midwife was also considered involved. In the remaining 12 cases, the consultant team alone was involved. In one, junior hospital staff failed to admit to hospital a primigravida with hypertension and proteinuria. By the time she was delivered hypertensive disease was severe and led to the intravascular coagulation defect which caused her death from severe bleeding and shock.

The consultant team was involved in another case in which labour was induced for hypertensive disease. Spontaneous delivery was followed by severe bleeding and a perineal haematoma, associated with disseminated intravascular coagulation. Delay with blood transfusion was considered an avoidable factor in her death and this was considered due in part to administrative failure, because blood for transfusion was not available in the hospital on a 24 hour basis. In addition, junior obstetric staff were involved for failing to inform the obstetric consultant of the patient's deteriorating condition; he became aware of her serious problem only during a routine hospital visit.

In 4 cases, blood loss appeared to have been underestimated and blood replacement was delayed or inadequate.

In 2 cases avoidable factors were considered to be associated with operative management and delivery. In one, persistent vaginal bleeding followed forceps delivery by a senior house officer and the consultant was not informed until the patient was *in extremis*. The large vaginal vault laceration from which she had actually been bleeding was then detected and sutured, but a haematoma developed in the broad ligament and laparotomy was performed to ligate the internal iliac artery and evacuate and pack the haematoma. Although the patient's condition improved dramatically, this was transient and she died later of cerebral anoxia. In the other patient, Caesarean section was required when attempted forceps delivery failed. Although the records in this case were poor, the patient apparently continued to bleed vaginally postpartum and a cervical tear had to be repaired under general anaesthesia. The postpartum bleeding led to severe shock and brain damage and she died some weeks later from bronchopneumonia.

The consultant team was also involved in four other cases. In one a patient who had a cervical suture removed at the 37th week of pregnancy, became dyspnoeic, cyanosed and collapsed in the second stage of labour. Amniotic fluid embolism was suspected. She was delivered by forceps and suffered severe postpartum haemorrhage. Continued vaginal haemorrhage could not be controlled despite manual compression of the uterus and a cervical tear was sutured. Although massive blood transfusion was given oliguria developed and she was transferred to a renal unit where septicaemia was diagnosed. Hysterectomy was performed the uterine wall being found to be full of micro-abscesses. Hyperpyrexia developed and the patient became decerebrate. Ultimately, ventilatory support was discontinued.

In another case labour was induced for severe hypertensive disease. Forceps delivery was followed by repeated bleeding into the episiotomy wound. Three successive haematomata had to be evacuated, the patient's haemoglobin level fell from 13 to 3.8 g/dl. During transfusion of 16 units of blood and other fluids administered without measurement of central venous pressure, the patient's blood pressure began to increase dangerously and she died from cerebral haemorrhage.

In another patient 3 days after a self administered overdose of 'aspirin' labour began and was associated with antepartum haemorrhage. Twins were delivered and the placenta which was adherent was manually removed. There was torrential postpartum haemorrhage, but with blood transfusion the patient's condition appeared to be satisfactory 6 hours after delivery. Further large volumes of blood and other fluids were transfused and the patient developed pulmonary oedema, followed by the 'shock lung' syndrome and died 2 weeks later.

In the remaining case a primigravida aged 22 was admitted to hospital because of severe hypertensive disease of pregnancy and vomiting. She developed jaundice and intrauterine fetal death occurred. Labour was induced by intravenous administration of Sytocinon followed later by amniotomy. An intravascular clotting defect developed and uterine activity became hypertonic. Labour progressed to forceps delivery to be followed by postpartum haemorrhage of 1600 ml. The Syntocinon infusion rate was increased and streptokinase and heparin were administered. Antibiotics, hydrocortisone, fibrinogen and fresh frozen plasma were given before delivery. There was further postpartum haemorrhage and although cardiac arrest occurred heart action was successfully restored. Postpartum bleeding continued and 5 hours later lacerations of the cervix and posterior fornix were found and sutured. Bleeding continued up to the time of her death, a total of 49 units of blood and 32 units of plasma having been administered. Treatment with heparin was continued until 8 hours before she finally died in her 5th cardiac arrest 6 days after delivery.

Addendum—Possible long-term effects of postpartum haemorrhage

In February 1978 the death occurred of a patient who 5 years earlier had had an exsanguinating postpartum haemorrhage. This was at home following a precipitate labour at 36 weeks in this, her second pregnancy, and she was entirely unattended. She was found by her husband when he returned from work and she was at first thought to be dead. The emergency obstetric service which was summoned arrived most expeditiously and was able to resuscitate her. Unfortunately, she suffered severe brain damage from the hypovolaemia and remained dumb and paraplegic. She was nursed at home and, despite most dedicated care by her family developed repeated urinary tract infections and renal calculi, ultimately dying of uraemia. No avoidable factors were considered present in her case. This case is not included in the enquiry but is mentioned to draw attention to the fact that occasionally death may occur long after the obstetric calamity basically responsible.

Summary and conclusions

1. Since the last report the total number of deaths and the mortality rate directly attributable to haemorrhage has increased. All of this has been due to an increase in deaths from postpartum haemorrhage. The number due to other causes in which haemorrhage contributed has decreased from 21 in 1973 − 75 to 14 in 1976 − 78. The proportion with avoidable factors in this report (65%) shows a reduction from the last report.

2. An unexplained feature of this report has been the increased number of deaths from postpartum haemorrhage in women of parity one, compared with previous reports. The number of deaths in this category in 1976 − 78 was 20 of a total of 27 (74%); in 1973 − 75 it was 6 of a total of 26 (23%).

3. In cases of placental abruption, the need for early and adequate blood transfusion, if necessary with group O rhesus negative blood, must again be stressed for 3 deaths were due to delayed or inadequate blood transfusion.

4. Caesarean section for placenta praevia should be carried out, or at least supervised by, a consultant wherever possible. Facilities for immediate operation and blood transfusions should be available in every consultant obstetric unit. Once again, attention is drawn to the danger of morbid adherence of the placenta to a uterine scar.

5. A blood coagulation disorder was a factor in 17 of the 40 deaths associated with haemorrhage. In 8 cases, amniotic fluid embolism was the suspected cause but in only 4 was the diagnosis confirmed histologically. In any type of haemorrhage in pregnancy the possibility of a coagulation disorder should always be considered. The advice of a haematologist should be obtained as soon as possible because inappropriate treatment, particularly with anti-coagulants, may worsen the condition and special expertise may be required in the management of coagulation failure from less common causes.

6. It is disappointing that the mortality rate from haemorrhage has not been reduced in the last 9 years. Too often has blood loss been underestimated, not reported early enough, or not properly investigated, diagnosed or managed. *'Too little, too late'*, seems too often to have been the fault in management. In several deaths, hysterectomy was delayed until shock had become irreversible. If bleeding cannot be controlled by manual compression of the uterus, direct compression of the aorta and treatment of any coagulation disorder, there should be no hesitation in opening the abdomen and either ligating the internal iliac arteries of performing hysterectomy. Such a procedure should be performed by an experienced obstetrician.

7. Realistic appraisal and replacement of blood loss is essential, and measurement of central venous pressure is the most effective means of monitoring the patient's changing condition, especially when bleeding has been severe and concealed, and extensive blood replacement required. It is recommended that each obstetric unit should have its own agreed procedure for the treatment of catastrophic haemorrhage. (See also the summaries in Chapters 8 and 9).

4. Pulmonary embolism

Forty-five deaths were coded to pulmonary embolism of which 14 occurred before delivery and 31 after delivery, 9 were after Caesarean section and 22 after vaginal delivery. All were coded ICD 673.2. Two additional deaths from pulmonary embolism followed abortion, one was coded to spontaneous abortion (ICD 634.6) and one to legal abortion (ICD 635.6). All of these 47 deaths have been included in the discussion and tables in this chapter. Deaths from pulmonary embolism have risen in 1976 – 78 compared with 38 in 1973 – 75, the increase being mainly in deaths after delivery. There were also 3 cases in which pulmonary embolism occurred but in which death was attributed to other causes. These are included in Chapters 3, 8 and 14.

There were no deaths from pulmonary embolism in association with ectopic pregnancy, hydatidiform mole or choriocarcinoma. One other death from pulmonary embolism is known to have occurred but cannot be included as no confidential enquiry form (MCW 97) was received. Death is known to have followed delivery and to have been associated with intravascular coagulation and a retained placenta. This compares with 4 deaths without confidential reports in 1973 – 75, 7 in 1970 – 72 and 11 in 1967 – 69.

Deaths from air embolism and amniotic fluid embolism are considered elsewhere (Chapters 13 and 10) and deaths from cerebral venous thrombosis are included in Chapters 13 or 14 as miscellaneous or associated deaths. Only 2 deaths which occurred 60 and 232 days respectively after vaginal delivery, would have been excluded under the international* definition of maternal death.

Table 4.1 compares deaths and Figure 4 death rates, from pulmonary embolism in this and previous reports. Death rates in 1976 – 78 appear to have increased compared with 1973 – 75, which had represented a marked fall compared with previous triennia.

Table 4.1: *Deaths from pulmonary embolism*

	1967 – 69	1970 – 72	1973 – 75	1976 – 78
Deaths after abortion	6*	11	3	2
Deaths during pregnancy	22	14	14	14
Deaths after vaginal delivery	36 (20)	30 (10)	15 (10)	22 (14.9)
Deaths after Caesarean section	18 (180)	17 (160)	6 (70)	9 (76.6)
Total	82	72	38	47

* Including one death after ectopic pregnancy
Rates per million vaginal deliveries or Caesarean sections given in parentheses

* See page 7

Tables 4.2 and 4.3 show the time intervals between delivery and fatal pulmonary embolism following vaginal delivery and Caesarean section in the 12 years 1967 to 1978.

Table 4.2: *Interval between delivery and pulmonary embolism following vaginal delivery, 1967 – 78*

	1967 – 69	1970 – 72	1973 – 75	1976 – 78	Total
Less than 24 hours	2	3	2	2	9
2 – 7 days	10	6	5	5	26
8 – 14 days	8	7	–	2	17
15 – 42 days	12	7	6	11	36
Over 42 days	4	7	2	2	15
Total	36	30	15	22	103

Table 4.3: *Interval between delivery and pulmonary embolism following Caesarean section, 1967 – 78*

	1967 – 69	1970 – 72	1973 – 75	1976 – 78	Total
Less than 24 hours	1	2	–	3	6
2 – 7 days	5	3	2	2	12
8 – 14 days	7	3	2	2	14
15 – 42 days	5	7	2	2	16
Over 42 days	–	2	–	–	2
Total	18	17	6	9	50

Figure 4 shows the death rate per million maternities for pulmonary embolism from 1952 – 1978.

Pulmonary embolism after abortion

One of the 2 deaths from pulmonary embolism followed spontaneous abortion at the 25th week in a 22 year old woman in her third pregnancy. She was well when discharged after 6 days but was re-admitted on the 10th day because of upper abdominal pain, thought to be due to pelvic infection. She appeared to recover with antibiotic treatment but she died suddenly on the 16th day. Autopsy confirmed the presence of a large embolus in the pulmonary artery but no obvious source was found except thrombus in the intra-uterine veins.

The other death occurred suddenly 3 days after vaginal termination combined with abdominal tubal ligation at 12 weeks gestation, in a 40 year old patient in her fourth pregnancy. A massive pulmonary embolus was confirmed at autopsy. The origin of the embolus was not sought.

The excess risk of an abdominal operation in conjunction with vaginal termination is well recognized. No avoidable factors were attributed to either of these cases.

Figure 4 *Death rate per million maternities from pulmonary embolism 1952-1978*

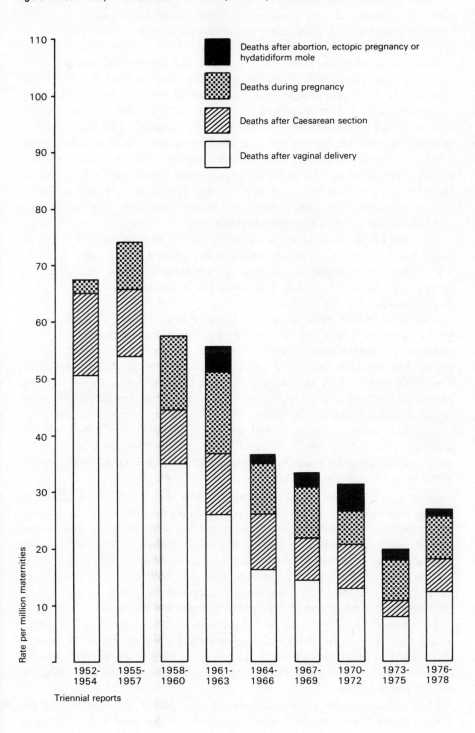

Deaths after abortion, ectopic pregnancy or hydatidiform mole

Deaths during pregnancy

Deaths after Caesarean section

Deaths after vaginal delivery

Rate per million maternities

Triennial reports

Pulmonary embolism during pregnancy

Death occurred from pulmonary embolism in pregnancy unexpectedly in 8 of the 14 women and with premonitory symptoms or signs in six.

Three patients had pulmonary embolism without preceding evidence of thrombosis. Fluid and electrolyte depletion may have predisposed to embolism in one woman who was admitted to hospital and required intravenous fluids for severe hyperemesis at 11 weeks gestation. She died suddenly at home 4 days after leaving hospital. Autopsy confirmed massive pulmonary embolism, with the appearance of thrombi suggesting an origin from veins of small calibre. The pelvic and leg veins showed no evidence of thrombosis. In a second patient in whom the clinical picture was confused by her history of recurrent chest infections sometimes associated with haemoptysis dehydration may also have played a part. She developed severe hyperemesis and intermittent dyspnoea. During the 11th week of pregnancy she was found dead in bed at home. Autopsy confirmed massive bilateral pulmonary embolism. The pelvic veins and the inferior vena cava contained thrombus.

The third patient complained of chest pain in the 30th week of her first pregnancy but no specific cause was found by her general practitioner. When he was visiting her at home 3 days later she suddenly collapsed and died. The general practitioner performed post-mortem Caesarean section but the child was stillborn.

Avoidable factors were considered to have been present in 6 cases. The patient alone was involved in 2 cases. In one, at approximately 20 weeks gestation the patient was referred to hospital for antenatal care but did not attend. She was later found in a collapsed state at home and died soon after. The other patient with an undiagnosed pregnancy was 45 years of age and developed both superficial thrombophlebitis and a deep vein thrombosis while in bed at home because of influenza. She died suddenly soon after admission to hospital having initially refused to go in. Autopsy confirmed bilateral superficial thrombophlebitis associated with severe varicose veins together with massive pulmonary embolus which appeared to have arisen from thrombi in the deep veins in the right leg.

General practitioners were considered to have been involved in 2 cases. In one the doctor did not suspect a patient's chest pain might be due to pulmonary embolism. A diagnosis which was confirmed at autopsy. The second general practitioner failed to make a diagnosis of deep vein thrombosis and gave only local treatment for superficial thrombophlebitis to a woman of 38 in the 7th week of her fourth pregnancy. She died suddenly 12 days later. At autopsy she was found to have a pulmonary embolus, one leg was grossly swollen and thrombus was found in both femoral and calf veins.

The general practitioner and consultant team were considered to be involved in one case. The patient who had a previous history of deep vein thrombosis complained of breathlessness at the 31st week of pregnancy and died without treatment from a confirmed pulmonary embolus arising from a thrombus in the left femoral vein.

The consultant team alone was involved in a case of an obese 39 year old woman in her third pregnancy who had severe varicose veins and a history of superficial phlebitis in previous pregnancies. Autopsy confirmed a large embolism in the pulmonary artery and thrombus in the proximal part of the left femoral vein.

Pulmonary embolism after vaginal delivery

Twenty-two deaths followed pulmonary embolism after vaginal delivery. Two deaths occurred more than 6 weeks after delivery and would be excluded under the international* definition of maternal death. There were 17 spontaneous deliveries, 3 forceps deliveries and 2 breech deliveries. Twelve of the women died suddenly and unexpectedly. The remaining 10 women had one or more warning symptoms or signs including those of superficial thrombophlebitis in 5, including one with dyspnoea and another with signs of pulmonary consolidation, deep vein thrombosis in 2, and suspected pulmonary embolism in 2. In one patient with chest pain, oral contraception was commenced 2 weeks after delivery and continued despite worsening symptoms. She died 60 days postpartum.

Four deaths followed operative procedures. In 2 of these, puerperal tubal ligation had been performed. In another, an infected perineum was resutured and in the fourth a ruptured uterus discovered after forceps delivery was repaired at laparotomy.

Avoidable factors were present in 9 cases. The patient alone was involved in 2, the general practitioner alone in 2, the consultant team in 4, and both the patient and the consultant team in one.

One patient was a diabetic whose poor co-operation made control difficult. She had a pulmonary embolism at the 28th week of pregnancy which was treated with heparin. Preterm labour occurred four days later. She died 40 days after delivery of massive pulmonary embolus, having co-operated poorly in her treatment. The other patient at fault failed to attend hospital until the 26th week of pregnancy despite severe hypertension. She died of pulmonary embolus 25 days after delivery. Earlier and regular attendance might have allowed different management and outcome in these cases.

The general practitioner was involved in 2 cases. One patient complained of chest pain 29 days after a normal delivery at term. He prescribed antibiotics attributing the chest pain to pulmonary infection. The patient died suddenly of a massive pulmonary embolus 4 days later. Another general practitioner was involved in a case where pain developed in the right leg 4 days after a normal confinement. The condition was treated as superficial thrombophlebitis until the diagnosis of pulmonary embolism became obvious 22 days later. Although she was immediately admitted to hospital cardiac arrest occurred soon after admission and she died despite pulmonary artery embolectomy.

The consultant team was involved in 4 instances. In one patient in whom the previous delivery had been by Caesarean section, labour was induced, the patient delivered with Kielland's forceps by a Senior House Officer and rupture of the uterus was discovered. Laparotomy was performed by a

* See page 7

Registrar and the uterus repaired. Three days later the patient collapsed and died of a massive pulmonary embolism. It was considered that too much responsibility had been delegated to the junior staff and that the consultant should have performed or at least supervised the laparotomy. In another case, a patient with severe varicose veins requested tubal ligation after the birth of her third child. This was performed 4 days after delivery and she died of massive pulmonary embolism 12 days later. The presence of varicose veins should have warned of an increased risk of thromboembolism. The risk may have been further increased by delaying the procedure until the fourth day after delivery. The consultant team was involved in another case in whom tubal ligation was performed 36 hours after delivery. The patient was kept in for 15 days after operation because of superficial thrombophlebitis. She was discharged home and died of a pulmonary embolus on the 40th post-operative day. Avoidable factors were also attributed to the consultant team in the death of a patient known to suffer from vascular anomalies of both lower limbs and previous deep vein thrombosis. In the present pregnancy she again developed deep vein thrombosis which was treated with anticoagulants which were discontinued at 31 weeks because of rectal bleeding. She was safely delivered at term following induction of labour. Three days after delivery she became dyspnoeic and shocked. No anticoagulant therapy was given because a diagnosis of cardiomyopathy was made as chest x-ray and ECG were normal. The fifth day after delivery she died of a massive pulmonary embolus, confirmed at autopsy, the thrombus having arisen in the pelvic veins. It was judged that the consultant team should have considered the diagnosis of pulmonary embolism as being most likely.

Finally, in one case avoidable factors were attributed to both the patient and to the consultant. This patient with social problems was admitted at 32 weeks gestation in her third pregnancy with a small antepartum haemorrhage. Her symptoms resolved and she was discharged home subsequently defaulting from the antenatal clinic. She was readmitted at 37 weeks in a collapsed state and a diagnosis of placental abruption was made. During induced labour the patient complained of chest pain. She was delivered following a rapid labour of a liveborn infant. There was no retroplacental clot. A diagnosis of pulmonary embolism was not made until the patient was seen by a physician and treatment with heparin initiated but the patient died. Autopsy confirmed pulmonary embolism with thrombus in the right deep femoral vein.

Pulmonary embolism after Caesarean section

There were 9 deaths from pulmonary embolism after Caesarean section, all of which occurred within 6 weeks of delivery.

Death followed Caesarean section performed before the onset of labour in 2 cases and during labour in 7 cases, 3 of which were induced. In 2 cases the clinical history or findings might have indicated an increased risk of pulmonary embolism. In one patient pleuritic pain and radiological evidence of a pleural effusion developed on the fifth post-operative day. No anticoagulant treatment was given and the patient died on the eighth day. Another patient developed a 'mild chest infection' with pyrexia on the second post-operative day and antibiotics were prescribed. Later that day she developed severe dyspnoea and cyanosis and died within 30 minutes.

Of the 9 deaths from pulmonary embolism after Caesarean section in 1976 – 78, only two had been resting in hospital for hypertensive disease of pregnancy before Caesarean section, in contrast to the 1973 – 75 triennium when 4 of 6 deaths from pulmonary embolism after Caesarean section were in women who had been resting in hospital for a considerable period of time before delivery.

Avoidable factors were considered to be present in 3 cases. In one patient the anaesthetist was involved when inhalation of vomit occurred during induction of anaesthesia for Caesarean section in labour for fetal distress. The consultant team was considered to be involved in a patient who had had a previous Caesarean section, when labour was induced by amniotomy and oxytocin infusion under epidural anaesthesia. After more than 11 hours in labour the uterus ruptured and sub-total hysterectomy was performed together with repair of the bladder. The patient developed pleuritic pain with radiological evidence of a pleural effusion on the fifth day but was not given anti-coagulants. Three days later she died of a massive pulmonary embolus, despite attempted pulmonary embolectomy. Finally, both the patient and the consultant team were considered to be involved in the case of a woman from Pakistan who had previously been delivered by Caesarean section because of osteomalacia. The consultant was considered involved because he had not arranged delivery by Caesarean section. The patient was involved because she had defaulted 7 times from the antenatal clinic and had refused operation for 6 hours. When the operation was performed a ruptured uterus was found and hysterectomy required and the patient died at home 12 days later from a pulmonary embolus. This was confirmed at autopsy.

Possible aetiological factors

Age and parity

Table 4.4 shows the total number of maternal deaths in relation to age for 1976 – 78 compared with 1967 – 75, and that this was similar to the expected number.

Table 4.4: *Number of maternal deaths from pulmonary embolism by age, 1976 – 78 compared with 1967 – 75*

Age	1967 – 75				1976 – 78	
	Total maternities	Number of deaths	Rate per million	†Expected deaths on basis of 1967 – 75 rates	Total maternities	Number of actual deaths
< 25	3,030,081	43	14.2	10	709,038	8
25 – 29	2,161,981	49	22.7	14	637,683	23
30 – 34	967,641	42	43.4	13	303,575	9
35 – 39	402,193	39	97.0	8	79,622	2
40 +	115,315	19	164.8	3	18,931	5
All ages	6,677,211	192	Total (by addition)	48	1,748,849	47

† For explanation of method of calculation see page 8

Table 4.5 shows the number of maternal deaths by parity in 1976 – 78 compared with 1967 – 75, and that there was no change compared with the previous triennia.

Table 4.5: *Number of maternal deaths from pulmonary embolism by parity*, 1976 – 78, compared with 1967 – 75*

Parity	1967 – 75				1976 – 78	
	Total maternities	Number of deaths	Rate per million	†Expected deaths on basis of 1967 – 75 rates	Total maternities	Number of actual deaths
1	2,680,166	56	20.9	16	747,409	17
2	2,230,024	43	19.3	12	643,922	10
3	998,707	32	32.0	7	233,388	9
4	417,750	22	52.7	4	76,247	8
5 +	350,564	37	105.5	5	47,885	3
Not stated	–	2	–	–	–	–
All	6,677,211	192	Total (by addition)	44	1,748,849	47

* For definition of parity see page 8
† For explanation of method of calculation see page 8

Table 4.6 shows the estimated rates per million maternities from pulmonary embolism by age and parity for 1970 – 78.

Table 4.6: *Maternal deaths due to pulmonary embolism by age and parity* (estimated rates per million maternities), 1970 – 78*

Age in years		Parity					
		1	2	3	4	5 +	All
Under 20	Number	8	–	–	–	–	8
	Rate	16.0	–	–	–	–	12.9
20 – 24	Number	13	7	2	1	–	23
	Rate	12.7	9.7	10.6	24.0	–	11.6
25 – 29	Number	18	22	9	8	3	60
	Rate	24.9	25.6	26.9	73.4	59.6	28.9
30 – 34	Number	7	7	7	2	6	29
	Rate	38.8	22.0	31.7	19.7	80.5	32.4
35 – 39	Number	–	1	7	5	9	22
	Rate	–	14.1	93.4	96.7	137.0	71.7
40 and over	Number	1	1	1	3	7	13
	Rate	109.4	78.4	65.7	223.8	222.1	158.5
All ages	Number	47	38	26	19	25	155
	Rate	18.9	18.1	30.9	59.8	108.0	25.9

* For definition of parity see page 8

Obesity

Sixteen of the 47 women who died from pulmonary embolism were 'overweight', defined as exceeding 75 kilograms in the last Report. A further 3 were described as 'obese' but their weights not recorded. Of the 16 women known to have been obese, 6 suffered from hypertensive disease of pregnancy. Nineteen patients were not overweight. There was no information about weight in 9 patients. Of the 38 women who died from pulmonary embolism and whose weight was known, 19 were obese.

Restricted activity

Restricted activity may have been a contributing factor in 7 cases as already described.

Sickle cell disease

No patient who died from pulmonary embolism in the 1976 – 78 triennium was known to have sickle cell disease.

Suppression of lactation by oestrogens

Of the 32 women who died after delivery (22 vaginal deliveries and 10 Caesarean sections), only 4 (12.5%) were known to have had lactation suppressed by oestrogens. One patient was known to have started on a combined oral contraceptive within 2 weeks of delivery.

No firm conclusions can be drawn from such small numbers. It is not known what proportion of women had lactation suppressed by oestrogens during the triennium. The known association between the administration of oestrogens and thromboembolic disease necessitates continuing caution in their use.

47

Post-mortem examinations

Post-mortem examinations were carried out in 45 of the 47 women who died from pulmonary embolism but the source of the embolism was not stated or not looked for in 12. In the 33 cases where the source of the embolism was investigated, it was thought to have arisen from thrombosed leg veins in 16 cases and from pelvic veins in 12 cases. In 4 other cases evidence of thrombus was found in both the pelvic and leg veins and also in the lower inferior vena cava in 3 of these. In one case the ovarian veins contained thrombus as well as the pelvic veins.

In one of the 2 cases where autopsy was not performed the patient died following pulmonary embolectomy but the site of origin of the thrombus was not determined. In the other case post-mortem examination was refused on religious grounds.

Evidence of the origin of the thrombotic process requires a careful search. Femoral or internal iliac vein thrombosis may spread from leg or pelvic veins.

Summary and conclusions

1. There were 47 deaths from pulmonary embolism, with firm pathological diagnosis in 46 including 2 deaths coded to abortion. One other death from pulmonary embolism is known to have occurred in this triennium. Two of the 47 deaths occurred more than 6 weeks after delivery and would be excluded under the international* definition of maternal death.

2. Of the 2 deaths after abortion, one occurred after spontaneous abortion and one after legal abortion combined with tubal ligation.

3. The number of deaths from pulmonary embolism during pregnancy was only one less than in the last triennium. Eight of the 14 deaths were sudden and unexpected.

4. There were 31 deaths after delivery in 1976 – 78 compared with 21 in 1973 – 75. Warning signs of thromboembolism were present in 10 of the 22 women delivered vaginally and in 3 of the 9 women delivered by Caesarean section. In the remaining 19 women, death occurred without warning.

5. Nineteen of the 47 women who died were obese; 6 of them also suffered from hypertensive diseases of pregnancy.

6. Eleven of the 22 women delivered vaginally and 4 of the 10 women delivered by Caesarean section, had been discharged from hospital before death.

7. None of the 47 women who died was known to have sickle cell disease.

8. Lactation was suppressed by oestrogens in 4 women who died after delivery. It is noteworthy that lactation was not suppressed in any of the women who died from pulmonary embolism following Caesarean section.

* see page 7

48

Although numbers are too small for firm conclusions, continued caution appears advisable.

9. The risk of thromboembolism increases with age, parity, obesity, previous thromboembolism, varicose veins, operative procedures such as Caesarean section. Since puerperal tubal ligation is an additional hazard it should be delayed.

10. Attention is again drawn to failure to consider the diagnosis of deep vein thrombosis or pulmonary embolism. The possibility should always be kept in mind that deep vein thrombosis can be recurrent and be present in association with superficial thrombophlebitis.

5. Abortion

Abortion was considered to be the direct cause of 14 deaths during 1976 – 78. Four deaths occurred in 1976 and 5 deaths in 1977 and 1978. This is the lowest number of abortion deaths since this series of reports started in 1952. Two deaths were due to spontaneous abortion (ICD 634), 8 deaths were due to legal abortion (ICD 635) and 4 deaths to illegal abortion (ICD 636). There were also 5 other true obstetric deaths due to complications of anaesthesia during operations for legal or spontaneous abortions, which are included in Chapter 8 and coded to ICD 668.

Table 5.1 and Figure 5 show the number of deaths from spontaneous, illegal and legal abortions from 1952 to 1978 inclusive and the rate per million maternities. Table 5.1 also shows the estimated rate per million conceptions since 1970.

Table 5.1: *Abortion deaths in triennial reports 1952 – 78, by type of abortion with estimated rates per million maternities and the estimated rates per million conceptions†, 1970 – 78*

Type of abortion	1952 – 1954	1955 – 1957	1958 – 1960	1961 – 1963	1964 – 1966	1967 – 1969	1970 – 1972	1973 – 1975	1976 – 1978
Illegal	108	91	82	77	98	74	38	10	4
Spontaneous	43	50	52	57	25	25	6	5	2
Legal*	2	–	1	5	10	18	37	14	8
Totals	153	141	135	139	133	117	81	29	14
Rates per million maternities	74.5	66.7	58.8	55.1	51.1	47.6	35.2	15.1	7.4
Rate per million conceptions	–	–	–	–	–	–	29.1	11.9	6.2

* Therapeutic abortion before April 1968
† Calculated as described in Chapter 1 page 8

The Abortion Act of 1967 effective from April 1968, made it compulsory to notify a legal abortion to the Chief Medical Officer of the Department of Health and Social Security or of the Welsh Office within 7 days of the operation. Statistics are published quarterly and annually by the Office of Population Censuses and Surveys and a commentary has been included since 1969 in the Annual Report of the Chief Medical Officer of the Department of Health and Social Security.

Figure 5 *Death rate per million maternities from abortion 1952-1978*

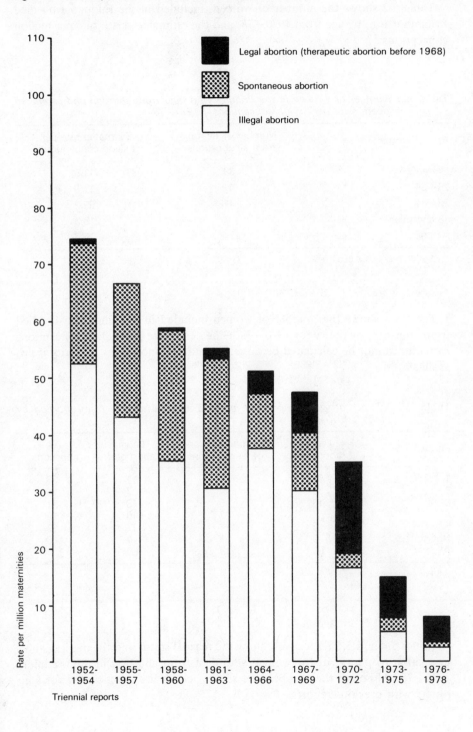

■ Legal abortion (therapeutic abortion before 1968)

▦ Spontaneous abortion

□ Illegal abortion

Table 5.1 and Figure 5 show deaths from illegal, spontaneous and legally induced abortion during the years 1952 to 1978 and are self explanatory. The effects of the Abortion Act on maternal mortality are apparent.

Table 5.2 shows the number of women, included in the Enquiry who died from abortion, by age from 1970 – 78, and the estimated death rate per million conceptions.

Table 5.2: *Number of women in the Enquiry who died from abortion and estimated death rates per million conceptions†, 1970 – 78*

Age of woman	Number of deaths from all abortions	Estimated rate per million conceptions
Under 25	39	11.9
25 – 34	41	11.6
35 – 44	41	68.2
45 and over	3	218.3
All ages	124	16.6

† See Chapter 1 page 8

Table 5.3 shows the number of women included in the Enquiry who died from abortion, by parity for 1970 – 78. (The death rate per million conceptions by parity cannot be calculated because the data of conceptions by parity is not available.)

Table 5.3: *Number of women included in the Enquiry who died from abortion by parity*, 1970 – 78*

Parity	Illegal abortions	Spontaneous and other abortions	Legal abortions	All abortions
1	14	1	11	26
2	9	–	7	16
3	13	5	13	31
4	7	2	10	19
5+	6	4	17	27
Not stated	3	1	1	5
All	52	13	59	124

* For definition of parity see page 8

Tables 5.4 and 5.5 respectively show the marital status and the marital status in relation to parity, of the women who died from abortion in the triennium 1976 – 78. Although the numbers are small these tables are included for continuity with previous reports.

Table 5.4: *Marital status of women who died from abortion, 1976 – 78*

Status	Illegal abortions	Spontaneous abortions	Legal abortions	All abortions
Married	2	1	6	9
Single, divorced or widowed	2	1	2	5
Total	4	2	8	14

Table 5.5: *Women who died from abortion: marital status in relationship to parity, 1976 – 78*

Status	Nulliparous	Multiparous	Total
Married	3	6	9
Single, divorced or widowed	3	2	5
Total	6	8	14

In the introduction to this report it has been stated that the causes assigned to deaths in this enquiry do not always correspond with those assigned by the Registrar General and this is so for deaths due to abortion. The numbers given in this and previous reports may therefore differ from those published by the Office of Population Censuses and Surveys.

Of the 14 deaths from abortion only one woman was non-Caucasian and she died from a spontaneous abortion.

Legal abortion

During the years 1976 – 78 there were 8 deaths due to legal abortion compared with 14 such deaths in 1973 – 75 and 37 in 1970 – 72. The fatality rate was 99.1 per million legal terminations during 1970 – 72, 29.8 in 1973 – 75 and 17.3 in 1976 – 78.

There were no deaths resulting from legal abortion in 1976; 4 in 1977 and 4 in 1978. These 8 terminations of pregnancy and the deaths all occurred in National Health Service hospitals.

Table 5.6 gives the details of length of gestation, age, parity and method of termination and mode of death for each mortality from legal abortion. This shows the high proportion of cases over 12 weeks gestation and over 40 years of age.

Table 5.6: *Deaths from legal abortion by duration, age, parity*, method of termination and mode of death — 1976 – 78*

Duration of pregnancy (weeks)	Age (years)	Parity*	Method of termination	Complications and mode of death
10	> 40	1	Dilatation and curettage	Incomplete termination; clostridial infection
11	> 40	4	Dilatation and curettage	Abdominal tubal ligation Pulmonary embolism
14	> 25	3	Extra amniotic prostaglandin and oxytocin	Ruptured uterus
14	< 20	1	Dilatation and aspiration	Uterus perforated. Intestinal obstruction Two laparotomy operations
14	> 40	8	Intra amniotic prostaglandin	Shock and pulmonary oedema. Cardiac arrest
15	< 20	1	Extra amniotic prostaglandin	Clostridial infection
16	> 40	5	Attempted dilatation and curettage, hysterectomy	Uterus perforated ⎫ during Intestine perforated ⎭ D & C Peritonitis
18	> 35	2	Intra amniotic prostaglandin and urea	Air embolism

* For definition of parity see page 8

Method of termination

Table 5.7 shows the number of terminations by method and the deaths resulting from them for 1976 – 78, when the death rate for all methods was 20 per million operations. The numbers of deaths by individual methods are too small for death rates to be considered useful, so that the rates for the 9 years 1970 – 78 have been calculated.

Table 5.7: *Legal abortion by type of operation 1970 – 78 and death rate per million operations (residents and non-residents)*

Type of operation	1976 – 78		1970 – 78		
	Number of operations 1976 – 78	Deaths in 1976 – 78	Number of operations 1970 – 78	Deaths in 1970 – 78	Death rate per million operations
Hysterotomy/hysterectomy[1]	4,817	1	53,084	16	301.4
D and C[2]	102,767	3	400,212	13	32.5
Vacuum aspiration only	265,445	–	683,600	9	13.2
Utus paste	63	–	3,974	8	2,013.1
Other methods[3]	31,143	4	82,149	13	158.2
Total	404,235	8	1,223,019	59	48.2

[1] Includes all procedures with mention of hysterectomy and/or hysterotomy

[2] Includes D and C with vacuum aspiration

[3] All methods not elsewhere classified (mainly medical) and 'not stated'.

Concurrent sterilization

There were two deaths following legal abortion in which the patient was sterilized at the same time as termination. One patient died from pulmonary embolism 3 days after a tubal ligation. The other patient died from carcinoma of the bowel 2 months after a laparoscopic sterilization, a fortuitous death.

Causes of death

Table 5.8: *Causes of death from legal abortion, 1976 – 78*

Cause of death	Number of cases
Sepsis	4
Cardiac arrest	1
Air embolism	1
Pulmonary embolism	1
Intestinal obstruction	1

Age

The age of women who died in 1976 – 78 is shown in Table 5.6.

Table 5.9: *Deaths from legal abortion by age, 1970 – 78 (residents only)*

Age (years)	Total operations 1970 – 78	Number of deaths† from legal abortion 1970 – 78	Death rate per million operations
< 16	22,248	2	89.9
16 – 19	122,942	7	56.9
20 – 24	151,448	6	39.6
25 – 29	121,947	8	65.6
30 – 34	99,354	6	60.4
35 – 39	75,366	11	146.0
40 +	38,989	12	307.8
Total	921,774	52	56.4

† *Note* Number of deaths from legal abortion for residents only included in the Enquiries

Parity

The parity of the women who died in 1976 – 78 is shown in Table 5.6.

55

Table 5.10: *Deaths from legal abortion by parity*, 1970 – 78 (residents only)*

Parity	Total operations 1970 – 78	Number of deaths† from legal abortion 1970 – 78	Death rate per million operations
1	446,631	10	22.4
2	109,470	6	54.8
3	166,021	12	72.3
4	106,651	9	84.4
5 +	88,323	15	169.8
Not stated	4,678	–	–
Total	921,774	52	56.4

† *Note* Number of deaths from legal abortion for residents only included in the Enquiries
* For definition of parity see page 8

Avoidable factors

One or more avoidable factors were present in 5 of the 7 deaths from legal abortion. In 4 of these it was attributed to the consultant team and in one instance to the consultant and the general practitioner. Three cases were worthy of mention.

Pregnancy was not detected by a registrar in a multiparous woman aged over 48 years with 10 weeks amenorrhoea. She was later admitted with acute retention of urine caused by an incarcerated retroverted gravid uterus. Termination of pregnancy per vaginam was attempted by the registrar and omentum was brought down into the vagina. At laparotomy for hysterectomy a perforation of small intestine was not detected. The subsequent appearance of free gas in the abdominal cavity on radiological examination was not considered to be an indication for laparotomy and the patient died of peritonitis.

A woman at 14 weeks gestation who had had 2 lower segment Caesarean sections was given extra-amniotic prostaglandin and an intra-venous infusion of Oxytocin. She was obese (weight 120 kg), and her blood pressure was 150/110 mm Hg. Abortion did not occur and after 3 days the treatment was repeated. After a further 4 days prostaglandin vaginal pessaries were introduced. Two days later, that is 9 days after the initial treatment, examination under general anaesthesia revealed a tear in the uterine fundus. The uterine rupture was repaired at laparotomy and she died 4 days later from acute generalized peritonitis.

A consultant extracted by vacuum suction the product of conception of 14 weeks gestation of a primigravid patient under 20 years. Three days later she was readmitted with abdominal pain and at laparotomy the uterus was shown to have been perforated and the small bowel ruptured. Paralytic ileus occurred and at laparotomy 10 days later a bowel resection was necessary. She died of intestinal obstruction.

There were also 4 other true deaths due to complications of anaesthesia during operations for legal abortions which are included in Chapter 8.

Legal abortion and associated diseases

There were 5 other deaths after legal abortion where the death was attributed to an associated cause rather than to the abortion, and are included in Chapter 14.

The cause of death in these cases were:

ICD 199	Carcinoma of Bowel	1
ICD 648.0 and 250.1 }	Bronchopneumonia and diabetes	1
ICD 648.2 and 282.5 }	Sickle cell disease	1
ICD 648.9 and 183 }	Sarcoma of ovary	1
ICD 648.9 and 570 }	Acute Hepatic Necrosis (unknown cause)	1

Illegal abortion

An avoidable factor has been attributed to the patient in all deaths from illegal abortion following the practice of previous reports.

Four deaths from illegal abortion were recorded, 2 in 1976 and one in each of 1977 and 1978. This continues the decline in this type of abortion mortality which started with 74 deaths in 1967 – 69 38 deaths in 1970 – 72 and 10 in 1973 – 75. (See Table 5.1).

Two were married and 2 were single women, all of Caucasian origin. One woman concealed her pregnancy and started to bleed heavily at the 16th week of gestation. Two weeks later she was admitted to hospital with defibrination syndrome and a haemoglobin concentration of 1.5 g/dl and pelvic sepsis. Another woman died at the 20th week of pregnancy from *E.Coli* and streptococcal septicaemia. Two women were found dead in their homes, 7 and 14 weeks pregnant respectively, one from air embolism and the other from septicaemia following the instillation of soap solution.

Spontaneous abortion

Two deaths occurred after spontaneous abortion in the period 1976 – 78 both being in 1976. This compares with 52 such deaths twenty years ago and 25 deaths ten years ago.

One patient who suffered from systemic lupus erythematosus died at home at the 20th week of pregnancy having had no antenatal care. The other woman died from pulmonary embolism 2 weeks after her abortion. (Included in Chapter 4).

There was no mention of an intrauterine contraceptive device being present in either patient.

There was also one other true death due to complications of anaesthesia during an operation for the removal of retained products following a spontaneous abortion. This case is included in Chapter 8.

Spontaneous abortion and associated diseases

There were 7 other deaths from spontaneous abortion where the death was attributed to an associated disease rather than to the abortion. They were all classified as indirect maternal deaths. The causes in these cases were:

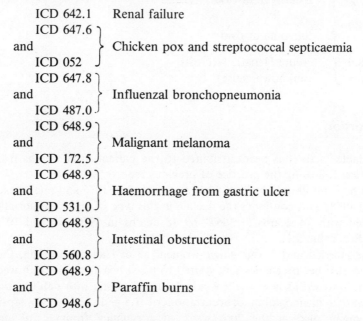

ICD 642.1   Renal failure

ICD 647.6
and   Chicken pox and streptococcal septicaemia
ICD 052

ICD 647.8
and   Influenzal bronchopneumonia
ICD 487.0

ICD 648.9
and   Malignant melanoma
ICD 172.5

ICD 648.9
and   Haemorrhage from gastric ulcer
ICD 531.0

ICD 648.9
and   Intestinal obstruction
ICD 560.8

ICD 648.9
and   Paraffin burns
ICD 948.6

Summary and conclusions

1. Deaths from all categories of abortion were considerably reduced in 1976 – 78 compared with the previous triennium.

2. There were 14 deaths from abortion in 1976 – 78 compared with 29 in 1973 – 75.

3. There were 4 deaths from illegal abortion in 1976 – 78 compared with 10 in 1973 – 75.

4. There were 8 deaths from legal abortion in 1976 – 78 compared with 14 in 1973 – 75. In both triennia there were 6 deaths in the second trimester of pregnancy.

5. There were 2 deaths from spontaneous abortion in 1976 – 78 compared with 5 in 1973 – 75.

6. Warning has been given in all reports since 1964 about the dangers of using Utus paste. For the first time since then no death was caused by this method; but it has had the highest mortality rate per 1,000 operations so it is regretted that this method is still in use.

6. Cardiac disease associated with pregnancy

Twenty one women died from cardiac disease associated with pregnancy during the period 1976−78, compared with 20 in 1973−75. Eleven women died from cardiac disease in 1973 and since then the annual number of deaths has been between 5 and 8.

In the 21 deaths now recorded there were 18 with acquired cardiac disease coded to ICD 648.6 and 3 with congenital abnormalities coded to ICD 648.5. They were all considered to be indirect maternal deaths.

Figure 6 shows the estimated death rates per million maternities for all cardiac disease subdivided between acquired and congenital disease. Data for congenital heart disease are not available prior to 1961, as up to that date they were included with other congenital abnormalities.

The numbers of maternal deaths associated with *acquired* cardiac disease in successive reports is:

1952−53	121	1967−69	34 (4)
1955−57	102	1970−72	33 (2)
1958−60	66	1973−75	16 (2)
1961−63	68	1976−78	18 (3)
1964−66	43		

Numbers in parentheses indicate the number that would be excluded under the international* definition of maternal deaths. This information is only available since 1967.

The numbers of maternal deaths associated with congenital cardiac disease since 1961, when they were first mentioned in these reports, is as follows:—

1961−63	13	1970−72	9
1964−66	7	1973−75	4
1967−69	15	1976−78	3

None of those occurring since 1967 would have been excluded under the international* definition of maternal deaths.

Age and parity

The distribution by age and parity of maternal deaths associated with all cardiac disease during 1976−78 is shown in Tables 6.1 and 6.2, and for

* See page 7

Figure 6 *Death rate per million maternities from cardiac disease 1952-1978*

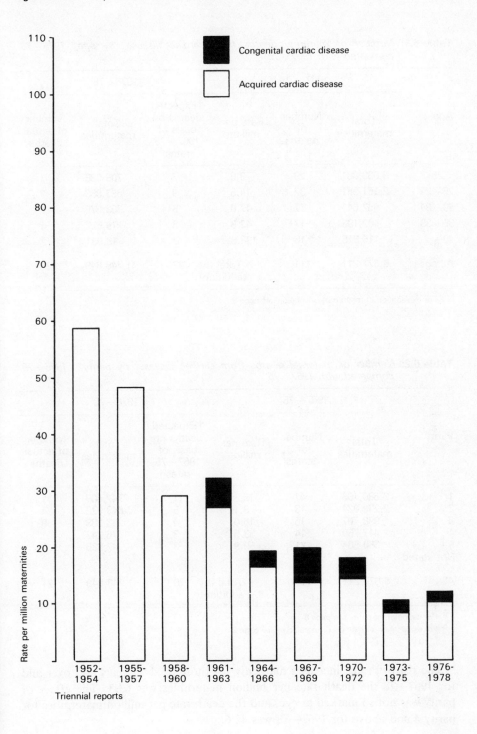

61

acquired and congenital disease in Tables 6.3 and 6.4 and compared with those in 1967 – 75.

Table 6.1: *Number of maternal deaths from cardiac disease, by age, 1976 – 78, compared with 1967 – 75*

Age	1967 – 75				1976 – 78	
	Total maternities	Number of deaths	Rate per million	†Expected deaths on basis of 1967 – 75 rates	Total maternities	Number of actual deaths
< 25	3,030,081	29	9.6	7	709,038	7
25 – 29	2,161,981	32	14.8	9	637,683	7
30 – 34	967,641	17	17.6	5	303,575	1
35 – 39	402,193	17	42.3	3	79,622	4
40 +	115,315	16	138.8	3	18,931	2
All ages	6,677,211	111	Total (by addition)	27	1,748,849	21

† For explanation of method of calculation see page 8

Table 6.2: *Number of maternal deaths from cardiac disease, by parity*, 1976 – 78, compared with 1967 – 75*

Parity	1967 – 75				1976 – 78	
	Total maternities	Number of deaths	Rate per million	†Expected deaths on basis of 1967 – 75 rates	Total maternities	Number of actual deaths
1	2,680,166	41	15.3	11	747,409	11
2	2,230,024	18	8.1	5	643,922	4
3	998,707	16	16.0	4	233,388	3
4	417,750	14	33.5	3	76,247	1
5 +	350,564	21	59.9	3	47,885	2
Not stated	–	1	–	–	–	–
All	6,677,211	111	Total (by addition)	26	1,748,849	21

* For definition of parity see page 8
† For explanation of method of calculation see page 8

The risk with age increases markedly for those aged 25 years and over and for 1967 – 78 the death rate per million maternities was 63.3. The effect of parity was not so marked as age, and the death rate per million maternities for parity 4 and above for 1967 – 78 was 42.6.

Table 6.3: *Number of maternal deaths from congenital and acquired cardiac disease, by age, 1967 – 78*

Age	Deaths from congenital cardiac disease				Deaths from acquired cardiac disease			
Years	1967 – 69	1970 – 72	1973 – 75	1976 – 78	1967 – 69	1970 – 72	1973 – 75	1976 – 78
< 25	10	2	1	1	5	8	3	6
25 – 29	2	5	2	2	12	6	5	5
30 – 34	–	2	1	–	9	4	1	1
35 – 39	2	–	–	–	2	9	4	4
40 +	1	–	–	–	6	6	3	2
All ages	15	9	4	3	34	33	16	18

Table 6.4: *Number of maternal deaths from congenital and acquired cardiac disease, by parity*, 1967 – 78*

Parity*	Deaths from congenital cardiac disease				Deaths from acquired heart disease			
	1967 – 69	1970 – 72	1973 – 75	1976 – 78	1967 – 69	1970 – 72	1973 – 75	1976 – 78
1	9	7	2	2	11	10	2	9
2	4	1	2	1	4	2	5	3
3	–	1	–	–	6	5	4	3
4	1	–	–	–	6	5	2	1
5 +	1	–	–	–	6	11	3	2
Not stated	–	–	–	–	1	–	–	–
All	15	9	4	3	34	33	16	18

* For definition of parity see page 8

Deaths due to acquired cardiac disease associated with pregnancy

Table 6.3 shows that 6 women died after the age of 35 years from acquired cardiac disease. This confirms the statement in previous reports that pregnant women with acquired disease are at special risk in the later years of reproductive life. When all the deaths from acquired disease for 1967 – 78 are considered this reveals a death rate for women aged 35 years and over to be 58.4 per million maternities, compared with 8.2 per million under 35 years.

Coronary artery disease caused the death of 7 women who were aged, respectively 22, 29, 32, 36, 36, 38 and 40 years. Analysis shows that the death rate from coronary heart disease per million maternities appears to be increasing, being 1.74, 2.60 and 4.0 in the triennia 1970 – 72, 1973 – 75 and 1976 – 78 respectively. The 22 year old woman weighed 83 kg, smoked 80 cigarettes daily and had a duodenal ulcer. She died in the 9th week of her first pregnancy of an acute myocarditis and post-mortem examination showed severe atheroma of the coronary arteries. A woman weighing 121 kg had an emergency Caesarean section for fetal distress and died 48 hours after the operation from coronary occlusion.

Cardiomyopathy was stated to be the cause of death of 5 women who were aged 17, 23, 23, 24 and 25. Two of these patients died three and a half months and four months after delivery respectively and so would be excluded under the international* definition of maternal mortality.

Acute and subacute bacterial endocarditis caused the death of 3 women. One of these is worthy of comment. The patient aged 28 who had had 2 spontaneous abortions, developed a septic finger, due to a staphylococcal infection at the 35th week of pregnancy. Erythromycin was prescribed but she did not take it. Four days later she developed a generalized macular rash with polyarthropathy. At the 37th week of pregnancy she went into spontaneous labour and had an easy vaginal delivery. Two days after delivery clubbing of the fingers was noticed with splinter haemorrhages. She developed cardiac failure and a loud murmur was heard. An emergency cardiac operation disclosed severe congenital and acquired cardiac disease. She died 36 hours after this operation. Mortality from staphylococcal endocarditis is high and in the rare instance of complicating pregnancy it carries a poor prognosis.

No other patients had cardiac surgery during pregnancy or the puerperium. One woman had previously been operated upon for a ventricular septal defect and she is included in the cases of congenital cardiac disease.

One patient developed an acute infective endocarditis and died 27 days after an emergency Caesarean section for cord prolapse. She had gram-negative septicaemia.

One woman who had had 2 previous Caesarean sections died at the age of 23 years from idiopathic pulmonary hypertension and associated heart disease two days after an emergency Caesarean section at the 32nd week of pregnancy.

Table 6.5: *Maternal deaths associated with acquired cardiac disease, 1970 – 78*

Triennial reports for the years	Rheumatic valvular disease	Bacterial endocarditis	Coronary artery disease	Other conditions including cardiomyopathies
1970 – 72	16	3	4	8
1973 – 75	3	5	5	3
1976 – 78	3	3	7	5

* See page 7

Table 6.5 shows the causes of death of patients who died from acquired cardiac disease from 1970 to 1978. During the 9 year period, 44 of the 67 deaths occurred after the 36th week of pregnancy, 7 before and 37 after delivery. Eight deaths occurred more than six weeks after delivery and would be excluded under the international* definition of maternal death. If the 59 remaining deaths are considered, 36 (61%) occurred after the 36th week of pregnancy showing the greater the risk to the woman the longer their pregnancies continued.

Deaths due to congenital cardiac malformations associated with pregnancy

Since the triennial report of 1961 – 63, maternal deaths due to congenital cardiac malformations have been recorded separately from acquired heart disease. Three patients with a congenital cardiac defect died during the years 1976 – 78, but since no post-mortem examination was carried out on any of them there must be doubt about the pathology. A summary is given of each case:

1. Ventricular septal defect closed surgically at age 14. In her first pregnancy she had acute cardiac failure. When pregnant for the second time she refused termination of pregnancy; labour started at the 37th week of pregnancy and a forceps delivery was performed when she was in early cardiac failure. She took her own discharge from hospital and died 4 weeks later on her way back to hospital.
2. Eisenmenger's defect in a woman aged 27 'so severe that death within a year seemed likely'. She had frequently been advised against pregnancy. Antepartum haemorrhage from a third degree placenta praevia necessitated an emergency classical Caesarean section by the consultant at the 38th week of pregnancy and the patient died the next day.
3. Eisenmenger's defect in a woman who had also had a patent ductus arteriosus closed when she was six months old. The ventricular septal defect found at that time was not corrected. She was advised not to become pregnant and subsequently refused termination of pregnancy. Labour was induced in the 39th week of her first pregnancy and with an epidural anaesthetic she was delivered of a fetus weighing 3.35 kg by vacuum extraction. She died 17 days postpartum.

Avoidable factors

There were one or more avoidable factors present in 4 of the 21 deaths associated with cardiac disease (19%). Three of these involved patients having an acquired cardiac lesion and one with a congenital cardiac defect.

In each instance the *patient alone* was responsible. Note that throughout these reports the refusal of a woman to accept advice for contraception and/or

* See page 7

termination of pregnancy has not yet been considered an avoidable factor. The presence of an avoidable factor in this context does not mean that death might have been avoided, rather it implies that the patient herself failed to obtain the high standard of care which was available and this may have contributed to the fatal outcome.

All 4 of these patients could have had the benefit of care by cardiologists, obstetricians and general practitioners and midwives. One woman had rheumatic fever when aged 9 and 13 years. In her second pregnancy, at the age of 41, she died at the 16th week of gestation without having consulted a doctor or midwife. Another died undelivered at the 32nd week of pregnancy having refused to go to hospital. A third patient, a grand multipara, refused any antenatal care and arrived in hospital in the second stage of labour. She would not stay in hospital after delivery and died at home in the company of her children, 17 days postpartum.

Finally a woman suffering from pulmonary hypertension took her own discharge from hospital and died 4 weeks later.

With one woman there was a language problem, which may have contributed to her death.

Summary and conclusions

1.   The total of deaths from cardiac disease associated with pregnancy, delivery and the puerperium during 1976 – 78 at 21 was substantially the same as during the previous triennium.

2.   Acquired and congenital cardiac disease maintained similar proportions.

3.   All women but one who died were of Caucasian origin.

4.   The greatest danger for women with acquired cardiac disease is after the 36th week of pregnancy, and particularly for women over the age of 35 years. Although the number of deaths from acquired cardiac disease due to rheumatic carditis has fallen, the number of deaths due to coronary artery disease has increased.

5.   There were no deaths attributable to anaesthesia associated with cardiac disease.

6.   Avoidable factors were present in 4 of the 21 maternal deaths and in each instance the patient was at fault.

7. Caesarean section

During the years 1976 – 78 there were 90 deaths connected with, but not necessarily due to, Caesarean section. Deaths so recorded in the triennia since 1952 are shown in Table 7.1 are as follows:—

Table 7.1: *Deaths connected with Caesarean section 1952 – 1978*

	Total	True maternal deaths	With an associated disease
1952 – 54	183		
1955 – 57	184		
1958 – 60	130		
1961 – 63	143		
1964 – 66	145		
1967 – 69	124		
1970 – 72	111	*84	*27
1973 – 75	81	61	20
1976 – 78	90	65	25

* *Note* Accurate information to classify these deaths into true and associated is not available before 1970

This total of 90 is made up of 65 *true* maternal deaths and 25 deaths caused by *associated* disease. There were 25 true maternal deaths in 1976, 20 in 1977 and 20 in 1978.

From the Hospital in-patient Enquiry (HIPE) conducted by the Department of Health and Social Security in England and Wales and the Office of Population Censuses and Surveys, an estimate may be made of the number of Caesarean section operations in National Health Service Hospitals in England and Wales. From this figure and from the deaths in the enquiry series, the fatality rate can be calculated as 0.8 per 1,000 Caesarean sections during the years 1976 – 78 which was the same as the 1973 – 75 rate (Table 7.2).

The increased number of deaths from Caesarean section compared with those reported to the Enquiry in the previous triennium, 1973 – 75 can probably be explained by two facts. The annual number of Caesarean sections performed had risen from about 33,000 in 1973 to 42,000 in 1978, an increase in the proportion of Caesarean sections in the total number of deliveries from 5.3 per cent in 1973 to 7.6 per cent in 1978. Also in the present triennium 1976 – 78, MCW 97 reports were completed on all the deaths associated with Caesarean section known to the Registrar General, whereas in 1973 – 75 six cases had to be excluded because no MCW 97 reports were received.

Table 7.2: *Estimated number of Caesarean sections performed, and estimated fatality rate per thousand Caesarean sections in NHS hospitals in England and Wales for each triennium, 1964 – 1978*

	1964 – 66	1967 – 69	1970 – 72	1973 – 75	1976 – 78
Total births in E & W	2,630,150	2,484,004	2,322,124	1,940,689	1,766,169
Estimated portion of Caesarean sections among all births %	3.4	4.0	4.4	5.2	6.7
Total maternities in NHS hospitals	1,807,552	1,926,308	2,000,612	1,799,980	1,689,670
Estimated number of Caesarean sections in all NHS hospital deliveries	88,290	99,480	103,310	101,410*	117,470
Percentage of maternities by Caesarean sections in NHS hospitals	4.9	5.2	5.2	5.6	7.0
Deaths after Caesarean section (True maternal and associated deaths from enquiry series)	145	124	111	81	90
Estimated fatality rate per thousand Caesarean sections	1.6	1.2	1.1	0.8	0.8

Note* The estimated number of Caesarean sections in NHS hospitals for the period 1973 – 75 has been altered since the last Report. A more direct method has been used in arriving at these estimates from HIPE data.

Immediate cause of death

Table 7.3 shows the distribution of the immediate cause of death related to Caesarean sections during 1976 – 78 separated into deaths with or without one or more avoidable factors. In this triennium the list of immediate cause of death correlates with the causes given in Appendix A, Table A1. This is partly because the anaesthetic deaths have their own code (ICD 668) and therefore, as described in Chapter 1, have not been coded to the indication for operation. Also in this triennium, except for three deaths included with the miscellaneous deaths in Chapter 13, all the true other deaths associated with Caesarean section have been classified to one of the main causes of death, hypertensive disease, haemorrhage, pulmonary embolism, amniotic fluid embolism or sepsis.

Table 7.3: *Distribution of immediate cause of death among Caesarean section deaths, 1976 – 78*

Immediate cause	Number of deaths with no avoidable factor	Number of deaths with avoidable factor	All deaths	
			Number	Percentage of total deaths
Haemorrhage	5	5	10	11%
Pulmonary embolism	5	4	9	10%
Sepsis	2	6	8	9%
Hypertensive diseases of pregnancy	5	7	12	13%
Anaesthesia	—	20	20	22%
Other true causes	5	1	6	7%
Associated diseases	23	2	25	28%
Total	45	45	90	100%

Table 7.4 compares the percentage distribution of all deaths after Caesarean section in 1976 – 78 classified according to the immediate cause of death, compared with the triennia since 1958. Table 7.5 shows the same groups of cases and the percentage with avoidable factors.

Table 7.4: *Percentage distribution of all deaths after Caesarean section, classified according to the immediate cause of death*

	1958 – 1960	1961 – 1963	1964 – 1966	1967 – 1969	1970 – 1972	1973 – 1975	1976 – 1978
Haemorrhage	43.8	23.8	14.5	11.3	7.2	9.9	11.1
Pulmonary embolism	20.9	20.3	18.6	14.5	15.3	7.4	10.0
Sepsis and paralytic ileus	17.7	13.3	17.9	8.9	14.4	9.9	8.9
Hypertensive diseases of pregnancy	6.9	9.8	4.1	4.8	13.5	14.8	13.3
Anaesthesia	3.8	13.3	13.8	25.8	17.2	21.0	22.2
Other causes (including associated diseases)	4.6	10.5	20.0	30.6	32.4	37.0	34.4
Total	100.0	100.0	99.9	100.0	100.0	100.0	99.9

Table 7.5: *Deaths after Caesarean section classified according to the immediate cause of death, percentage with avoidable factors*

	1958–1960	1961–1963	1964–1966	1967–1969	1970–1972	1973–1975	1976–1978
Haemorrhage	56.2	26.5	42.8	64.3	50.0	87.5	50.0
Pulmonary embolism	7.4	17.2	7.4	16.7	23.5	33.3	33.3
Sepsis and paralytic ileus	26.1	15.8	26.9	63.6	62.5	87.5	75.0
Hypertensive diseases of pregnancy	–	15.3	83.3	66.7	66.7	66.7	58.3
Anaesthesia	20.0	42.1	60.0	75.0	78.9	94.1	100.0
Other causes (including associated disease)	–	13.3	13.8	15.8	22.2	30.0	12.9
Total	31.5	22.4	27.6	53.5	45.9	60.5	50.0

Table 7.6 shows the number of maternal deaths by age and parity connected with Caesarean section 1970–78 and the death rates per million maternities. It indicates the increasing risk of death with age and parity.

Table 7.6: *Number of maternal deaths by age and parity* connected with Caesarean section 1970–78 and rates per million maternities*

Age Years	1	2	3	Parity 4	5+	Not stated	All	Rates per million maternities
< 20	12	–	1	–	–	–	13	76.8
20–24	36	12	4	–	–	1	53	98.2
25–29	44	27	9	4	1	–	85	133.3
30–34	18	18	13	10	8	2	69	227.3
35–39	11	4	7	5	11	–	38	477.3
40–44	2	3	3	5	10	–	23	1,319.5
45 and over	–	1	–	–	–	–	1	66.7
Total	123	65	37	24	30	3	282	161.2
Rates per million maternities	164.6	100.9	158.5	314.8	626.5	–	161.2	

* For definition of parity see page 8

Haemorrhage

In the years 1961–78 deaths from haemorrhage after Caesarean section were as follows:—

Years	1961 – 63	1964 – 66	1967 – 69	1970 – 72	1973 – 75	1976 – 78
Number of deaths	34	21	14	8	8	10

In 5 of the 10 cases in which haemorrhage was the immediate cause of death one or more *avoidable* factors were considered to play an important role in the ensuing death. In this series there was no common factor in these cases. Five women had a hysterectomy performed in an attempt to stop the haemorrhage.

In several instances time-wasting procedures such as packing the uterus were carried out. For example a woman had had 3 previous Caesarean sections for cephalo-pelvic disproportion and she had an antepartum haemorrhage from a type III anterior placenta praevia in her 4th pregnancy. A registrar opened the uterus through a classical incision and was faced with torrential haemorrhage when separating the placenta. The uterus was packed and a blood transfusion of 18 units was given. Ten hours later a hysterectomy was performed. Direct aortic compression during and after the section would have halted the bleeding, a simple and effective method of stopping uterine haemorrhage.

Pulmonary embolism

In the years 1961 – 78 deaths from pulmonary embolism after Caesarean section were as follows:—

Years	1961 – 63	1964 – 66	1967 – 69	1970 – 72	1973 – 75	1976 – 78
Number of deaths	29	27	18	17	6	9

One or more avoidable factors were considered present in 3 of the 9 deaths. One death from pulmonary embolism occurred during labour and an emergency Caesarean section was carried out with the delivery of a living baby at the 35th week of pregnancy. The membranes had ruptured 10 days before the onset of labour and the patient had been kept in bed and then developed deep vein thrombosis.

Sepsis

In the years 1961 – 78 deaths from sepsis after Caesarean section were as follows:

Years	1961 – 63	1964 – 66	1967 – 69	1970 – 72	1973 – 75	1976 – 78
Number of deaths	19	26	11	16	8	8

One or more avoidable factors were considered present in 6 of the 8 deaths caused by sepsis after Caesarean section, mostly attributable to poor post-operative management and including one instance of injury to the small intestine which was not noticed by the consultant at the operation.

71

One patient had chronic urinary tract infection caused by a renal staghorn calculus. She refused admission to hospital, but had a Caesarean section by a very junior registrar as an emergency. She had been poorly supervised by the consultant during pregnancy, labour and puerperium.

Seven of the deaths occurred after an emergency section and one after an elective Caesarean section.

One death occurred after a Caesarean section for fetal distress. Severe haemorrhage occurred at the time of operation when the registrar left the patient to attend to the twins who in fact were stillborn. Paediatric help should have been available when twins were expected. This was regarded as an administrative failure. The mother later died of sepsis.

Hypertensive diseases of pregnancy

During the years 1961 – 78 deaths from hypertensive diseases of pregnancy associated with Caesarean section were as follows:—

Years	1961 – 63	1964 – 66	1967 – 69	1970 – 72	1973 – 75	1976 – 78
Number of deaths	14	6	6	15	12	12

Eighteen women died following Caesarean section for hypertensive diseases of pregnancy, 15 with pre-eclampsia and 3 with eclampsia and 12 of the deaths were coded as being directly due to these diseases. Of these, 7 had one or more avoidable factors caused by delay in treatment incurred by the patient, general practitioner or consultant staff.

A patient (who had had hypertensive disease in a previous pregnancy) was attended at home by her general practitioner developed fulminating hypertension with albuminuria. She was found comatose at home was admitted to hospital and died of a cerebral haemorrhage after Caesarean section and delivery of a live child. If she had been under observation in a consultant unit the severity of the hypertensive disease would have been recognized and treatment given.

Anaesthesia

Deaths associated with anaesthesia for Caesarean section during the years 1961 – 78 were as follows:—

Years	1961 – 63	1964 – 66	1967 – 69	1970 – 72	1973 – 75	1976 – 78
Number of deaths	19	20	35	19	17	20

Deaths associated with anaesthesia for Caesarean section continue to be a cause of anxiety especially because *all* the 20 deaths in 1976 – 78 were considered to have one or more avoidable factors. These cases are discussed more fully in Chapter 8.

Other causes

There were 31 other causes of death associated with Caesarean section during the years 1976 – 78. Six of these had a *true* maternal cause of death, three dying from amniotic fluid embolism and three from miscellaneous causes. Of these one case was considered to have an avoidable factor.

Twenty-five women died from an associated disease of which 3 were considered to have one or more avoidable factors. Seventeen were considered to be indirect deaths, including 7 cases of cardiac disease and 8 were fortuitous. The causes of death were as follows:—

<table>
<tr><td colspan="3">Indirect Deaths</td></tr>
<tr><td colspan="3">All, ICD code 648 + Additional code</td></tr>
<tr><td>200.1</td><td>Lymphosarcoma of breast</td><td>1</td></tr>
<tr><td>227.8</td><td>{ Phaeochromocytoma extra-adrenal site</td><td>1</td></tr>
<tr><td>345.5</td><td>Temporal lobe epilepsy</td><td>1</td></tr>
<tr><td>395.0</td><td>Aortic stenosis*</td><td>1</td></tr>
<tr><td>410</td><td>Acute myocardial infarction</td><td>1</td></tr>
<tr><td>414</td><td>Chronic ischaemic heart disease</td><td>2</td></tr>
<tr><td>416.0</td><td>Idiopathic pulmonary hypertension</td><td>1</td></tr>
<tr><td>421.0</td><td>Acute infective endo-carditis</td><td>1</td></tr>
<tr><td>446.4</td><td>Thrombotic thrombocy-topenic purpura*</td><td>1</td></tr>
<tr><td>493</td><td>Asthma</td><td>2</td></tr>
<tr><td>518.1</td><td>Interstitial emphysema (pulmonary)</td><td>1</td></tr>
<tr><td>551.3</td><td>Diaphragmatic hernia, with gangrene</td><td>1</td></tr>
<tr><td>674.0</td><td>Cerebrovascular disorder in puerperium</td><td>1</td></tr>
<tr><td>745.4</td><td>Eisenmenger's defect</td><td>1</td></tr>
<tr><td>{ 991.0
  E901.0</td><td>{ Accidental death—
Exposure* while suffering from puerperal depression</td><td>1</td></tr>
</table>

<table>
<tr><td colspan="3">Fortuitous Deaths</td></tr>
<tr><td colspan="3">ICD Code</td></tr>
<tr><td>191</td><td>Malignant neoplasm of brain</td><td>1*
2 } 3</td></tr>
<tr><td>225</td><td>Benign neoplasm of cerebral meninges—causing cerebral oedema</td><td>1</td></tr>
<tr><td>323</td><td>Viral encephalitis*</td><td>1</td></tr>
<tr><td>430</td><td>Subarachnoid haemorrhage</td><td>1</td></tr>
<tr><td>431</td><td>Intracerebral haemorrhage</td><td>1</td></tr>
<tr><td>560.2</td><td>Volvulus*</td><td>1</td></tr>
</table>

Six of these women died more than 42 days after delivery and so would be excluded from the international† definition of maternal death. (Cases marked with an asterisk*).

† See page 7

Indications for operation

These were so varied and multiple that it is impossible to produce a table listing the principal reason for performing Caesarean section.

Status of the operator

The status of the operator who performed the Caesarean section, compared with that in previous reports, was as follows:—

	1967 – 69	1970 – 72	1973 – 75	1978 – 78
Consultant obstetrician	56	37	22	32
Senior registrar	42	12	8	9
Registrar		47	42	41
Senior house officer	7	8	7	4
House surgeon				
SHO with Consultant				1
Senior hospital medical officer	2	–	2	1
General practitioner obstetrician				
Clinical assistant				
SHO with Registrar	–	–	–	1
Not stated	17	7	–	1
	124	111	81	90

Avoidable factors

One or more avoidable factors were considered present in 45 (50%) of the total of 90 deaths connected with Caesarean section during the years 1976 – 78 which is less than in the previous triennium (1973 – 75) but higher than the preceding reports from 1961 as indicated here:

Years	1961 – 63	1964 – 66	1967 – 69	1970 – 72	1973 – 75	1976 – 78
Avoidable factors %	22.4	27.6	43.5	45.9	60.5	50

Sixty-five per cent of the true deaths connected with Caesarean section were considered to have one or more avoidable factors compared with 12% of the deaths with associated diseases. The responsibility for the avoidable factors was allocated as follows:—

Consultant obstetrician alone	11
Anaesthetist alone	17
General practitioner alone	4

Patient alone	2
Consultant obstetrician and anaesthetist	3
Consultant obstetrician and general practitioner	3
Consultant obstetrician and anaesthetist and patient	1
Consultant obstetrician and patient	3
Consultant physician	1
	45

It is important to stress that in many instances Caesarean section was delegated to relatively junior staff when the difficulties were complex both for the operator and for the anaesthetist. An allocation of responsibility for an avoidable factor to the consultant obstetrician or anaesthetist refers to all the medical staff under the overall supervision of the consultant.

Summary and conclusions

1. The number of deaths connected with Caesarean section during 1976 – 78 in England and Wales was 90. Sixty five were true maternal deaths and 25 were associated deaths.

2. The fatality rate for Caesarean section in 1976 – 78 was 0.8 per 1,000 Caesarean sections performed in National Health Service hospitals, the same rate as in 1973 – 75 to be compared with 1.1 in 1970 – 72 and 1.2 in 1967 – 69.

3. There were 10 deaths from haemorrhage in 1976 – 78 compared with 8 in each of the triennia 1973 – 75 and 1970 – 72.
   There were 9 deaths from pulmonary embolism in 1976 – 78 compared with 6 in 1973 – 75 and 17 in 1970 – 72.
   There were 8 deaths from sepsis in 1976 – 78 compared with 8 in 1973 – 75 and 16 in 1970 – 72.

4. The number of deaths from anaesthesia associated with Caesarean section showed no improvement for there were 20 such deaths during 1976 – 78 all with one or more avoidable factors compared with 17 in 1973 – 75 and 19 in 1970 – 72.

5. The percentage of one or more avoidable factors considered to be present in all the deaths connected with Caesarean section has remained at about the same level being 50% in 1976 – 78, 60.5% in 1973 – 75, 45.9% in 1970 – 72 and 43.5% in 1967 – 69.

Addendum

Post-mortem Caesarean section.
Six cases were recorded during 1976 – 78, compared with 7 in 1973 – 75.
The causes of maternal death were as follows: —

1. Amniotic fluid embolism (2).
2. Pulmonary embolism.
3. Inhalation of gastric contents.
4. Essential hypertension and diabetes.
5. Accidental burning in fire at home.

Four infants were stillborn and 2 died within 1 week of delivery.

None of these cases is recorded in the tables or in the summary and conclusions of this Chapter.

8. Deaths associated with anaesthesia

There were 40 deaths associated with anaesthesia in this triennium, 12 in 1976, 19 in 1977 and 9 in 1978. In 30 cases death was directly attributable to anaesthesia and in 10 anaesthesia played a part in morbidity leading to death. Avoidable factors were judged to have existed in all but 2 cases.

The estimated mortality rate per million maternities was 17.2 compared to 16.1 in the past two triennia. The percentage among the true maternal deaths was 13.2 the same as in 1973 – 1975 as shown in Table 8.1.

Table 8.1: *Deaths associated with anaesthesia: estimated rate per million maternities and percentage of true maternal deaths, 1964 – 78*

	1964 – 66	1967 – 69	1970 – 72	1973 – 75	1976 – 78
Number of deaths directly associated with anaesthesia	50	50	37	31	30
Rate per million maternities	19.2	20.3	16.1	16.1	17.2
Percentage of true maternal deaths due to anaesthesia	8.7	10.9	10.4	13.2	13.2

In the previous Reports deaths associated with anaesthesia have been classified to the condition necessitating the operative procedure for which the anaesthetic was given. However, ICD 9 for the first time contains a specific code 668 for 'Complications of the administration of anaesthetic or other sedation in labour and delivery'. Therefore in the present Report, deaths associated with anaesthesia administered during pregnancy, labour and delivery (see Chapter 1) have been classified according to the complication of the anaesthetic which caused death. See Table 8.2 and Table A1 in the Appendix A.

Table 8.2: *Deaths associated with anaesthesia, complications of the anaesthetic causing death during pregnancy, labour or delivery*

ICD Code	Complications	Number of deaths
668.0	*Pulmonary complications* of anaesthesia	
	(i) Inhalation of stomach contents	5 ⎫
	(ii) Inhalation of stomach contents and endotracheal tube wrongly placed (E876.3)	9 ⎬ 16
	(iii) Pulmonary oedema and endotracheal tube wrongly placed (E876.3)	1 ⎪
	(iv) Respiratory arrest	1 ⎭
668.1	*Cardiac complications of anaesthesia*	
	(i) Cardiac arrest	4 ⎫
	(ii) Cardiac arrest and failure of apparatus (E874.0)	1 ⎬ 6
	(iii) Cardiac failure and endotracheal tube wrongly placed (E876.3)	1 ⎭
668.2	*Central nervous system complications* of anaesthesia	
	(i) Cerebral anoxia	2 ⎫
	(ii) Cerebral anoxia and endotracheal tube wrongly placed (E876.3)	5 ⎬ 7
668.2	*Other complications* of anaesthesia Gas embolism and failure of apparatus (E874.0)	1
Total		30

The operative procedures for which anaesthesia was required are given in Table 8.3.

Table 8.3: *Deaths associated with anaesthesia: operative procedures for which anaesthetic was given*

Operation	Indication	Number of deaths
Vacuum aspiration	Legal termination	2
Evacuation of uterus, D and C	(i) Incomplete abortion	1 ⎫ 2
	(ii) Legal termination	1 ⎭
Hysterectomy	Legal termination	1
Pain relief in labour	Labour	1
Forceps delivery	Persistent occipito-posterior	1
Proposed emergency Caesarean section (Died during induction of anaesthesia)	Prolonged labour	1
Elective Caesarean section	(i) Pre-eclampsia	1 ⎫
	(ii) Placenta praevia	1 ⎬ 3
	(iii) Pre-eclampsia Disproportion	1 ⎭
Emergency Caesarean section	(i) Failed induction of labour	1 ⎫
	(ii) Disproportion	6 ⎪
	(iii) Fetal distress	4 ⎬ 17
	(iv) Prolonged labour	5 ⎪
	(v) Antepartum haemorrhage	1 ⎭
Manual removal of placenta	Retained placenta	1
Laparotomy	Ectopic pregnancy	1

Of the 24 women whose pregnancies had progressed beyond the 28th week, 2 died undelivered. There were no stillbirths. Of the 22 live births, three died in the early neonatal period and one before the end of the first month.

Anaesthetic causes of death

As in the last report deaths associated with anaesthesia are classified according to factors which initiated the events leading to death. This will aid continuity and simplify comparison. It must be stressed however that no comparison of statistical validity can be produced since it is not possible to provide rates in a statistical sense. The overall number of anaesthetics which have been given for any particular obstetrical complication is not ascertainable.

Cross referencing of patients with more than one anaesthetic factor operating has not been generally attempted since all are multifactorial and the information would have no practical use, but some histories fall naturally into two or more groups. The paragraph headings are:—

Inhalation of stomach contents
Difficulty with endotracheal intubation
Misuse of drugs
Accidents with apparatus
Epidural analgesia
Miscellaneous causes
Contributing anaesthetic factors
Status of anaesthetist
Failure of administrative arrangements
Monitoring during anaesthesia and operation

In this triennium most of the MCW 97 reports have been more fully completed than formerly and the anaesthetic contributions to death have been rather easier to discern but it will be noted where any doubts remain. The exact sequence of events may not have been completely clear in some instances but the attribution of 'with avoidable factors' has not been in doubt. It must be borne in mind that the reports are scrutinized remotely with hindsight and from an elitist standpoint, with the assumption that there should always have been faultless anaesthetists and obstetricians with skilled help working in ideal circumstances, so that few cases are classed as being without avoidable factors. Nevertheless these reports, if they are to have any value must highlight shortcomings in management as an educational contribution to safety in anaesthesia for childbirth.

Inhalation of stomach contents

Eleven patients (2 in 1976, 8 in 1977 and 1 in 1978) inhaled regurgitated gastric contents and died as a direct result of it while in 3 others this was most probably the event leading to death.

Nine patients developed Mendelson's syndrome (acid aspiration syndrome) and succumbed over periods varying from one death in the operating theatre, to one at 37 days postpartum. Six of these patients died within 2 days. Two patients developed bronchopneumonia and died in 7 and 11 days respectively.

Of the 3 uncertain cases one patient was reported to have aspirated regurgitated fluid during attempts at intubation and when intubation succeeded, inflation of the lungs proved to be impossible. On balance, it seems to be equally likely to have been an oesophageal rather than an endotracheal intubation. The second patient, having a Caesarean section, had a difficult intubation in which it was reported that cricoid pressure was released to give oxygen between attempts. She died from a pulmonary embolus on the 16th postpartum day having had a wound dehiscence and second anaesthetic on the 7th day. Anaesthesia was contributory to death. The third of these patients, a known asthmatic, had a lower segment Caesarean section under epidural analgesia. The administration of ergometrine intravenously caused vomiting with aspiration and intractable bronchospasm from which she died. Intravenous ergometrine should if possible be avoided in conscious patients because of the vomiting and other effects such as headache which it causes. Its side effects can be minimized by giving small doses slowly. It should be remembered that the recommended intra-venous dose is one quarter of that given intramuscularly or subcutaneously. Since the patient was asthmatic anaesthesia was classed as contributory, and the case is included in Chapter 14.

Of the 9 patients who developed Mendelson's syndrome 4 were reported to have routine medication with 'mist.mag trisil.', it was not given in 2 and there is no note in the remainder. Cricoid pressure was applied, obviously ineffectively in 5 patients and was not noted in the other 4. One patient who died from the acid aspiration syndrome on the 11th postpartum day was reported to have had 9 doses of antacid during labour.

Of the two patients with bronchopneumonia, one inhaled stomach contents during attempts at endotracheal intubation in the course of anaesthesia for a lower segment Caesarean section for cephalopelvic disproportion while in labour. Both cricoid pressure and antacids were used but assistance was casual and unskilled. The other patient regurgitated and aspirated when having a suction termination of pregnancy under a combination of epidural analgesia and heavy sedation administered by her obstetrician. This is noted under 'epidural'.

It is clear from the records of these patients that death was not the result of single errors or omissions but was most usually a combination of inexperience, low general standards of care in labour and in the operating theatre and poor administrative practices, in the form of unskilled assistance or isolation from fully equipped hospitals.

Difficulty with endotracheal intubation

In 16 patients difficulty with endotracheal intubation was the factor leading to death, 3 in 1976, 7 in 1977 and 6 in 1978. In only one of these was there any considerable doubt.

80

In 7 patients death resulted from inhalation of stomach contents and these have already been noted. In the 9 remaining patients the endotracheal tube was placed in the oesophagus, certainly in 6 and most probably in 3, death in these patients being due to the immediate or late effects of asphyxia.

In 3 other patients difficulty with intubation contributed to death. One patient was plethoric Hb 16 g/dl, hypertensive and had chronic bronchitis. Her operation was characterized by cyanosis and respiratory difficulty, due to endobronchial placement of the endotracheal tube. Neuromscular conduction could not be restored with neostigmine at the end of operation. The patient was then sent from an isolated obstetric unit to a district general hospital by ambulance and had a cardiac arrest in transit. This appears to have been an example of 'neostigmine resistant curarisation' which was unrecognised but no nerve stimulator was used. The second patient was asthmatic yet the recorded notes were not those of bronchospasm during operation but more probably those of oesophageal intubation. The remaining case in which difficulty with intubation contributed to death was that of the patient who died on the 16th day following Caesarean section already noted under 'inhalation of stomach contents'.

Multiple attempts at intubation by more than one anaesthetist are characteristic of some of these cases. In one patient for example there were persistent attempts at intubation, successively by a registrar and a consultant and eventually she had a tracheostomy. It was known that vomitus was inhaled during the first attempts, the patient was allowed to wake up to await the consultant and anaesthetized again while further unsuccessful attempts at oral and nasal intubation were made. General anaesthesia was then maintained by facepiece for tracheostomy and through the tracheostomy tube for operation. Although tracheostomy might have been a rational anticipatory procedure in view of the earlier inhalation of vomitus, the tube was removed at the end of operation despite further vomiting, only to be reinserted when her general condition had deteriorated to an irreversible state. There was not attempt at artifical ventilation or other intensive care.

It would be pointless to relate other equally disturbing histories because the message is clear. An adequate drill for difficult intubation must be taught and put into practice by all who give anaesthetics for obstetric patients. The apparent obsession that an endotracheal tube must be passed even if to do so requires successive attempts by anaesthetists in ascending order of seniority is not rational and in this triennium led to death. Anaesthesia to a depth classified by Guedel as III(i) or III(ii) prevents vomiting even without an endotracheal tube and is less harmful to the neonate than having no mother.

Misuse of drugs

Four patients, 3 in 1977 and 1 in 1978, died from misuse of drugs. In 2 this was from ignorance while in the third, misuse was probably accidental. The fourth consisted of the use of ergometrine intravenously in a conscious patient and this case is noted under the section on epidural analgesia and on inhalation of stomach contents.

The first of these patients was a short (140 cm) dark skinned woman who had a spontaneous abortion at mid-term and who was anaesthetized for removal of retained products of conception. Pre-medication was with papaveretum and hyoscine and anaesthesia was induced with diazepam 15 mg, pentazocine 30 mg and *Althesin* 1.5 ml given intravenously. Maintenance was with intermittent increments of *Althesin* while the patient was breathing air spontaneously. After about forty minutes she apparently stopped breathing and had irreversible cardiac arrest. The second patient was another dark skinned woman who was anaesthetized for suction termination of pregnancy. Pre-medication was with papaveretum 20 mg and hyoscine 0.4 mg and the obstetrician used 15 ml of 0.5 per cent lignocaine with 1 in 200,000 adrenalin for paravervical block. This was acceptable technique, but in addition she was also given diazepam 20 mg and methohexitone 80 mg intravenously followed by increments of methohexitone. After operation she had respiratory arrest followed by cardiac arrest and she died some days later from the effects of cerebral anoxia. These two patients had overdoses of respiratory depressant drugs, their skin colour masking cyanosis so that hypoxia passed unnoticed.

The third patient had an uneventful prolonged anaesthetic for termination of pregnancy. A small dose of tubocurarine had been given at the beginning and atropine 1.2 mg and neostigmine 5 mg were given for reversal of the neuromuscular block when the patient awakened. Bradycardia leading to intractable cardiac arrest occurred almost at once. Some doubts existed as to the identity of the drugs used so that this is classed as a doubtful case.

Accidents with apparatus

Two patients died as a result of accidents with apparatus.

In the first case the patient was given a general anaesthetic for an emergency Caesarean section. The patient who was dark skinned, was underventilated as a result of a technical error with a ventilator and suffered an irreversible cardiac failure from hypoxia.

The second death was due to pulmonary barotrauma with extensive cardiac and cerebral gas embolism which occurred at the end of a Caesarean section. A consultant was teaching his junior to use ether with the Oxford vaporizer (EMO) with an Oxford Inflating Bellows and Ruben valve. When the consultant left, the junior turned on a high gas flow from the Boyle's machine through the bellows jamming the Ruben valve in the inflating position to produce gross over inflation of the lungs and gas embolization.

Epidural analgesia

Four deaths occurred in the triennium in association with epidural analgesia, two in 1977 and two in 1978.

To one patient, an obstetrician, acting as his own anaesthetist administered 20 ml of 0.5 per cent bupivacaine epidurally for suction termination of pregnancy at 8 weeks. Pre-medication was with papaveretum (20 mg) and hyoscine (0.4 mg) and during operation when the patient became restless she was given diazepam (10 mg i.v.). She vomited and aspirated some gastric contents. An anaesthetist was called and resuscitated the patient but she succumbed from aspiration bronchopneumonia ten days later.

Another patient, who was asthmatic, was given 10 ml of 0.5 per cent bupivacaine (plain) epidurally for pain in labour at term. The registrar anaesthetist then returned to base hospital five miles distant. Over about 20 minutes there was a steady fall in blood pressure from 150/100 mm Hg to 80 mm Hg systolic and an inexperienced senior house officer gave *Dextran 70*. The patient developed bronchospasm and despite treatment by a consultant anaesthetist who was called, she finally had cardiac arrest. The primary cause was judged to have been subarachnoid block and there was an administrative failure in that no one who could deal with complications of epidural analgesia remained immediately available to the patient.

Of the other two deaths occurring in association with the use of epidural analgesia one has been noted in the sections on inhalation of stomach contents and misuse of drugs, the other had a general anaesthetic for Caesarean section following a trial of labour under epidural analgesia. This patient had inadequate post-operative supervision and had a cardiac arrest in the ward, dying a week later from the effects of cerebral anoxia.

Epidural analgesia should only be used by those properly trained to manage it and who are fully aware of the effects and hazards of regional blocks to mid-thoracic levels. It should never be used when a properly trained anaesthetist cannot be immediately available if required.

Miscellaneous causes

Nine deaths are noted in this section, 7 occurred in 1976 and 2 in 1977. They were all classed as having avoidable factors although this was doubtfully so in two patients.

Five of the patients died from haemorrhage in widely differing anaesthetic circumstances. Their histories are worthy of note in that they show fundamental deficiencies in anaesthetic practice, in awareness and in assessment and management of patients who are bleeding.

One patient delivered spontaneously and normally but continued to bleed following the third stage. After about four hours, during which bleeding continued, examination under anaesthesia was planned, the patient then having a rapid and feeble pulse and a blood pressure of 95/50 mm Hg. No plasma volume expander had been given and blood could not be obtained because the patient had a rare antibody. Before and during general anaesthesia for examination, 1,500 ml plasma was given by the anaesthetist but cardiac arrest occurred at the end of an inconclusive exploration of the genital tract. This was judged to be an example of inadequately treated haemorrhage, the severity of blood loss not being recognized.

One patient died from haemorrhagic shock from postpartum haemorrhage following delivery under epidural analgesia and pudendal block. This 120 kg dark skinned patient is reported to have received all the blood transfused, some six units, into subcutaneous tissues. The inexperienced team were acting beyond their competence.

A third death from haemorrhage occurred from the improper management of continued postpartum bleeding by a junior anaesthetist and inexperienced junior obstetrician. No expert anaesthetic or obstetric help was summoned until the patient was *in extremis*. It is clear from the report that no one on the team had adequate knowledge of the management of bleeding.

The fourth death occurred during hysterectomy for postpartum haemorrhage. The anaesthetists appeared to be so pre-occupied in trying unsuccessfully to pass an endotracheal tube in this patient who had a tempero-mandibular joint ankylosis that she bled to death without their active intervention.

The fifth patient also died during the course of hysterectomy for postpartum haemorrhage caused by a ruptured uterus. An entirely inadequate quantity of blood was transfused for severe blood volume deficiency during a one and a half hour operation and the patient succumbed. It is clear that there were no estimations of blood pressure, pulse rate or central venous pressures and that the anaesthetist did not appreciate the gravity of the patient's condition.

Management of severe blood loss is fundamental to any doctor's training and it is unlikely that any one of these five patients would have died had the haemorrhage been due to other trauma. It should not have to be said that all the normal management methods in haemorrhage of observation, estimation of blood pressure, blood loss, pulse rate, respiration, central venous pressure and active blood volume replacement should be available and in use in all delivery suites.

One patient died 120 days after a post-operative asphyxial episode. Anaesthesia was for vaginal termination of an early pregnancy, under cervical block and general anaesthesia. The patient never recovered from anaesthesia and asphyxiated while in the recovery area with an anaesthetic face mask to a Magill circuit strapped in place. This case would be excluded under the international* definition of maternal death.

One patient who was dark skinned had a cardiac arrest following elective lower segment Caesarean section. This was judged to be due to chronic hypoxia most probably due to failure to ventilate the lungs.

A patient with cardiomegaly, hypertension and diabetes died during induction of anaesthesia by a registrar anaesthetist. She was to have an elective lower segment Caesarean section. Cardiac arrest occurred, probably from hypoxia during intubation but the history is too complicated to give in detail and is classed as being doubtful with respect to avoidable factors. The registrar should have had senior assistance.

The last patient in this section had an incomplete spontaneous abortion at 22 weeks gestation and was anaesthetized for continued bleeding. Recovery was not rapid and an overload of intravenous fluids was given with resulting pulmonary oedema. She died 10 days later in the intensive care unit from gastro-intestinal haemorrhage. The history was much too inadequate to be able to judge what contribution to the death was made by the anaesthetic.

* See page 7

84

Contributing anaesthetic factors

All of the case histories in which anaesthesia was contributory to the fatal outcome have already been noted in the preceding paragraphs. Those cases in which anaesthesia made a contribution are 10 in number and the operative procedures for which an anaesthetic was given are listed in Table 8.4, and the main causes of death in Table 8.5.

Status of anaesthetist

No note has been made in this chapter on the status of the anaesthetist except where the information might have had some significance. It seemed to be more useful to indicate only where skill and knowledge were inadequate for the task in hand, in order to stress that obstetric anaesthetic deaths although relatively unchanged in numbers for this triennium are not at an irreduceable minimum.

Avoidable factors due to failure of administrative arrangements

In many of the case histories given in this chapter anaesthetists in first contact with the patients who died were lacking in adequate knowledge and skill. This should not be accepted as an inevitable feature of staffing of the NHS. It is seen particularly clearly in some of the cases of death from difficulties in endotracheal intubation and from haemorrhage that the individuals concerned were deficient in ordinary medical knowledge. No matter how skilled technically junior doctors might appear to be it is in difficult situations that basic deficiencies in their medical training appear and in the cases documented led to death. Before being placed in the position of first anaesthetic contact with obstetric patients junior doctors should have had adequate supervised surgical emergency and obstetric experience. It is apparent too that the less knowledgeable the anaesthetist the more likely is he (she) to accept inadequate conditions and ancillary help, thereby compounding the dangers.

Table 8.4: *Operative procedures for which anaesthetic was given where anaesthetic factors contributed to death*

Operation	Indication	Number of deaths
Evacuation of uterus	Spontaneous abortion	1
Emergency Caesarean section	(i) Fetal distress (ii) Prolonged labour	2 } 3 1
Proposed elective Caesarean section (PM Caesarean section performed)	Diabetes and hypertension	1
Removal of retained placenta	Retained placenta and haemorrhage	1

Table 8.4: *continued*

Operation	Indication	Number of deaths
Suture of cervical tear	Cervical tear and haemorrhage	1
Laparotomy	Vaginal lacerations and haemorrhage	1
Subtotal hysterectomy	Cervical tear and haemorrhage	1
Hysterectomy	Ruptured uterus and haemorrhage	1

Table 8.5: *Main causes of death in cases where anaesthetic factors contributed to death*

ICD		Number of deaths
I True maternal deaths		
665.1	Rupture of uterus during and after labour	1
666.0	Third-stage haemorrhage (associated with retained placenta)	1
666.1	Other immediate postpartum haemorrhage	3
673.2	Obstetrical blood-clot embolism (pulmonary)	1
II Indirect maternal deaths		
648.0	Other conditions of the mother complicating pregnancy—diabetes mellitus	1
648.9 531.0 }	Other conditions of the mother complicating pregnancy—haemorrhage from gastric ulcer	1
648.9 493 }	Other conditions of the mother complicating pregnancy—asthma	2

Monitoring during operation

As in the last report it is necessary to reiterate that anaesthesia for obstetric emergencies cannot be safely and efficiently given without the normal observations and measurements afforded to surgical patients. There are no situations of such emergency in obstetrics that the pulse rate and blood pressure cannot be estimated and trends of change followed.

It follows that all consultant obstetric departments should be equipped with the means of monitoring pulse, blood pressure, electrocardiogram and central venous pressure; of testing neuromuscular conduction and of maintaining mechanical ventilation of the lungs.

Summary and conclusions

1. Of the 40 deaths associated with anaesthesia all but 2 were judged to have had avoidable factors. Since most of these were attributable to combinations of lack of knowledge, inexperience, low general standards of care in labour

and poor administrative practices there is a need to review the anaesthetic services in maternity units with the aims of providing better trained anaesthetists and of ensuring that the administrative arrangements are inherently safe for patients.

2. Eleven patients died from the inhalation of stomach contents, 9 of these dying from Mendelson's syndrome.

Of those with Mendelson's syndrome 4 only appeared to have had routine antacid therapy yet it must be remember that this routine is merely a back-up to prevention of vomiting and regurgitation of stomach contents during anaesthesia. For this, experienced anaesthetists with skilled assistance are required.

3. Sixteen deaths were associated with difficulties in endotracheal intubation.

It is recommended that every obstetric unit should have an established drill for dealing with this complication of anaesthesia so that patients are not needlessly lost. This proposal should be examined by all anaesthetists who give anaesthetics for obstetrics.

4. Four deaths in this triennium were associated with epidural analgesia.

Although the method is technically easy and is easily taught, it is unwise to use it in obstetrics until the anaesthetist has had comprehensive experience of it in surgical practice.

It is also unsafe to use epidural analgesia in labour and for delivery if the anaesthetist is not immediately available to attend to the patient. This is not a counsel of perfection, simply a recommendation to transfer the same level of anaesthetic care to obstetric patients as that regarded as being essential in surgical practice.

5. There were 5 deaths from haemorrhage to which anaesthetic factors contributed.

It might possibly save lives if anaesthetists and obstetricians jointly devised a drill for managing this complication in their units.

6. The detection of cyanosis is difficult in dark skinned patients and this contributed to 5 deaths. Whatever the patient's skin colour the effects of hypoxia are detectable by following the blood pressure and pulse rate and by watching for other signs of altered autonomic activity. As in the last triennial report it is unfortunately necessary to emphasize that it is most unwise to anaesthetize patients without at least making use of such simple and elementary observations.

9. Ruptured uterus

Rupture of the uterus caused 14 maternal deaths. Eleven of these are classified under ICD 665.1 and 3 under 665.0. Five other deaths are known to be associated with rupture of the uterus but have not been counted in this chapter because 3 resulted from pulmonary embolism and are included in Chapter 4, one from legal abortion with sepsis included in Chapters 5 and 12, and one from eclampsia, included in Chapter 2. Seven babies were born alive although one died in the neonatal period, 5 were stillborn, including stillborn twins one of which was abnormal. One other baby died with its mother. In the remaining 2 cases, there were maternal and fetal deaths both at the 16th week of pregnancy from spontaneous uterine rupture in one and rupture of a myomectomy scar in the other.

Uterine rupture is described under three categories:

i. *Scar rupture*, following a previous operation, usually Caesarean section.

ii. *Traumatic rupture*, occurring from the use of instruments or intra-uterine manipulation. It is sometimes difficult to determine whether spontaneous rupture may have taken place before these procedures.

iii. *Spontaneous rupture*, which may occur as a result of strong uterine contractions with or without oxytocic agents or obstructed labour. The cause is often obscure, but it may sometimes be due to unrecognized trauma at a previous abortion or delivery.

Comparison with previous reports. Table 9.1 shows that there has been an apparent increase in the total number of deaths. For the first time since 1961 – 63, the triennium under review shows an increase in the overall rate per million maternities. However, the data must be interpreted with caution when such small numbers are involved.

Table 9.1: *Categories of uterine rupture, 1955 – 78*

	1955/57	1961/63	1964/66	1967/69	1970/72	1973/75	1976/78
Scar rupture	4	6	3	2	3	1	2
Traumatic rupture	21	13	12	9	2	3	6
Spontaneous rupture—without oxytocin	8	19	15	3 ⎱ 8	1 ⎱ 8	4 ⎱ 7	3 ⎱ 6
with oxytocin	–	–	–	5 ⎰ Ø	7 ⎰ X	3 ⎰	3 ⎰
Total	33	38	30	19	13	11	14
Rates per million maternities	15.6	15.1	11.5	7.7	5.7	5.7	8.0

Ø 2 Buccal 'Pitocin'
X 2 Buccal 'Pitocin'

Uterine scar rupture occurred in 2 cases.

In the first case, a 41 year old primigravida at the 16th week of pregnancy was given rectal suppositories by her practitioner when she complained of abdominal pain and constipation at a domiciliary visit. Myomectomy had been performed 10 months before. Two hours later the patient collapsed and was dead when the practitioner returned. At autopsy the peritoneal cavity contained 1,500 ml blood and the uterus was enlarged to 16 weeks gestation. The fundus of the uterus was 'paper-thin' and showed a crescentic rupture on the left side with herniation of placental tissue.

In the second case, a 34 year old woman was admitted at term in spontaneous labour in her 6th pregnancy. Six years before she had been delivered by Caesarean section for placenta praevia, but had subsequently had a vaginal delivery. Labour lasted less than 4 hours and a large infant, 4.64 kg was delivered after a second stage of only 11 minutes. There was a postpartum haemorrhage of 1,700 ml and despite blood replacement the patient's condition worsened. The uterus was well contracted. At laparotomy 4 hours after delivery, a tear 13 cm long, was found running transversely through the lower segment and extending outwards on the right. Hysterectomy was not performed because the patient by this time was moribund.

Two other women died following rupture of previous Caesarean section scars, but neither are counted as deaths from ruptured uterus because both died from pulmonary embolism and are described in Chapter 4.

Traumatic rupture occurred in 6 cases.

All were multiparous and had assisted vaginal deliveries. Five were delivered by forceps following intravenous oxytocin infusion and in one, breech extraction of an abnormal second twin was attempted after internal podalic version.

One Asian patient had her labour induced for pre-eclampsia in her 4th pregnancy, although the fetal head was 'free'. Although only 1.48 m tall and known to have a small pelvis, she had had 3 previous vaginal deliveries, including one stillborn breech. Amniotomy was performed and intravenous oxytocin infusion and epidural anaesthesia commenced. The fetal heart rate and unterine contractions were monitored. Despite episodes of fetal bradycardia, labour continued for over 12 hours and a stillborn fetus was delivered with Kielland's forceps. There was a postpartum haemorrhage of 800 ml and exploration of the uterus revealed rupture of the lower segment with extension into the broad ligament. A large haemoperitoneum was found and the blood loss was so profuse that death occurred during laparotomy performed without anaesthesia in this moribund patient.

A woman in her third pregnancy had labour induced at 42 weeks by amniotomy and intravenous oxytocin infusion. After 12 hours of labour, a 4.0 kg infant was delivered with Kielland's forceps. The placenta was manually removed, a cervical laceration repaired and 2 units of blood transfused. The patient's condition deteriorated, uterine rupture was suspected and laparotomy revealed a tear in the right side of the uterus. She died 4 hours after delivery following subtotal hysterectomy and blood transfusion.

Another woman in her second pregnancy was admitted with spontaneous rupture of the membranes before term and had labour accelerated by intravenous infusion of oxytocin. The presentation was breech. Forceps were used to complete easy delivery of an infant weighing 2.4 kg, in unexpectedly poor condition. Retroplacental clot was found and there was postpartum haemorrhage of 600 ml. Bleeding continued despite intravenous oxytocin infused in high dosage and exploration revealed uterine rupture. Laparotomy was delayed because of problems with anaesthesia. Despite hysterectomy, the patient died from uncontrollable bleeding with a large haematoma in the left broad ligament.

A 34 year old woman with twins in her third pregnancy suffered intrauterine death of one twin at 33 weeks. Spontaneous rupture of the membranes occurred at 34 weeks, the liquor being meconium-stained. Labour progressed to spontaneous delivery of a macerated first twin after 2 hours. Progress ceased and radiological examination requested by an obstetric registrar, summoned from another hospital 10 miles away, revealed an abnormal fetus. The consultant advised internal podalic version and breech extraction under general anaesthetic but delivery proved impossible. Uterine rupture was suspected when there was vaginal bleeding and deterioration in the patient's condition. At laparotomy, there was a litre of blood and a grossly abnormal, dead fetus in the abdominal cavity. The consultant performed hysterectomy and ligation of the internal iliac vessels, but bleeding from the vaginal vault and the lateral pelvic wall proved uncontrollable. The patient died after 3 hours in the operating theatre.

A 33 year old woman in her 6th pregnancy, described as 'independently minded', originally requested home birth but reluctantly accepted hospital delivery because she had a history of pyelonephritis. Although polyhydramnios developed at 39 weeks and the consultant advised admission for induction of labour, the patient was unwilling and was not admitted until the membranes ruptured spontaneously 22 days after term. Although labour was accelerated by intravenous oxytocin infusion the second stage was prolonged for over 2 hours. Forceps delivery proved very difficult, strong traction being required to deliver a 4.6 kg infant. Immediately after delivery, the patient developed respiratory arrest, became restless, violent and then died. At autopsy, several litres of blood were found in the abdomen, and there was a tear in the uterus just above the cervix, posteriorly and on the right, 10 cm long.

A 39 year old woman in her 8th pregnancy was found at term to have a hydrocephalic fetus with spina bifida. She had delivered an infant with this anomaly in a previous pregnancy. Labour was induced by intravenous oxytocin infusion after epidural anaesthesia; amniotomy was subsequently performed. After 12 hours, when the cervix was almost fully dilated, the patient collapsed. Epidural anaesthesia was 'topped up', oxytocin infusion stopped and the infant delivered by forceps after perforation of the head. Bleeding continued after delivery of the placenta and exploration revealed rupture of the posterior lower segment extending to the right cornu. Subtotal hysterectomy was performed by the consultant but bleeding continued and 9 hours later a second laparotomy had to be performed the right internal iliac artery ligated and the pelvis packed. Blood replacement of 9 units was considered adequate, cardiac arrest occurred and the patient died 5 hours after the second operation. At autopsy death was found to be due to congestive heart failure with extensive pulmonary oedema.

In another woman in whom traumatic uterine rupture occurred, death was assigned to hypertensive disease of pregnancy as she succumbed from cerebral haemorrhage following eclampsia despite an initially normal blood pressure. A stillborn infant was delivered by vacuum extraction after 17 hours labour. After a succession of postpartum complications, including disseminated intravascular coagulation, inhalation of vomit and pulmonary oedema, persistent vaginal bleeding led to examination under anaesthesia, at which an annular tear was found in the lower segment. Although this was repaired at immediate laparotomy, the patient died during the operation.

Spontaneous rupture occurred in 6 cases.

Three of these were associated with the administration of oxytocic drugs to multiparous patients. Oxytocin was used in two and oral prostaglandin E_2 in one. In each, the progress of cervical dilation was rapid and delivery precipitous. In each case, there was severe postpartum haemorrhage and the patient died despite massive blood transfusions and hysterectomy being performed or attempted.

The fourth patient, a 27 year old Bengali woman presented at a hospital casualty department complaining of abdominal pain and amenorrhoea of 14 weeks duration. She was suffering from shock, her condition worsened rapidly and she died despite resuscitative measures. Autopsy revealed extensive haemoperitoneum due to rupture of the fundus of the uterus with partial extrusion of the uterine contents, a fetal arm protruding from the amniotic sac. There was no evidence of interference or of previous uterine surgery.

In the fifth case a para 2, uterine rupture occurred without warning. After spontaneous onset of labour 10 days before term, an infant weighing 3.5 kg was delivered normally after a labour of 3½ hours. Blood loss in the normal third stage was 300 ml. Twenty minutes after expulsion of the placenta, there was massive postpartum haemorrhage. A subclavian vein catheter was inserted, because of difficulty in cannulating arm veins, but despite blood transfusion, cardiac arrest occurred. Endotracheal intubation was carried out and external cardiac message restored the heart beat. At laparotomy, a 7.5 cm long rupture was found in the uterus at the junction of the upper and lower uterine segments and subtotal hysterectomy was performed. Thirteen units of blood were administered and although the patient seemed initially to improve, she collapsed 4 hours later. Continuing intra-abdominal bleeding was not confirmed at a second laparotomy and intra-thoracic bleeding was suspected. Thoracotomy revealed severe bleeding from a hole at the junction of the left subclavian and innominate veins which was repaired with difficulty. A further 11 units of blood were transfused but the patient died and autopsy confirmed extensive mediastinal haemorrhage.

In the sixth case, a woman in her second pregnancy died suddenly at home in the 29th week. She had been in good health at several hospital antenatal examinations. At autopsy, the abdomen contained 2 litres of blood and blood clot, the fetus within the amniotic sac and the placenta, all lying free. The uterus showed a transverse tear in the fundus, 13 cm long. Histological examination revealed that placental villi had penetrated the full thickness of the uterine wall. There was no evidence of interference or of previous uterine surgery. Two other women died following spontaneous uterine rupture. One is counted in Chapter 4, and the other in both Chapters 5 and 12.

Avoidable factors

Avoidable factors were considered to be present in 11 of the 14 cases. In one, the patient herself was considered to be involved, because she refused to be admitted for induction of labour and subsequently required difficult forceps delivery of a large infant, 22 days after term. In one case the general practitioner was involved.

In each of the other 9 cases, the consultant team was considered to be implicated.

In 4, there was delay in diagnosis or treatment which proved fatal. In one of these it was also considered that the severity of bleeding had been underestimated and that too much responsibility had been delegated to inexperienced junior medical staff.

In 5 cases the avoidable factors were considered to be associated with poor clinical management.

In 2 other cases there was administrative failure in that adequate facilities for blood transfusion were not available to the consultant team.

Other clinical features

Tables 9.2 and 9.3 show the number of women by age and parity who died from rupture of the uterus. The figures show that the overall increase in incidence was not due to an increased number of patients of higher parity, but there was an increase in deaths in the younger age groups 25 to 34 in 1976 – 78 compared with the rates for 1967 – 75.

As in the last report, severe postpartum haemorrhage was a common feature, occurring in 9 of the 14 patients. The true incidence was even higher because 3 patients died undelivered and postpartum haemorrhage therefore occurred in 9 of the 11 patients with ruptured uterus who were delivered. Oxytocic drugs (including prostaglandins) were used in 8 women, all multiparous. Oxytocin was given to induce labour in 5 and to accelerate slow labour in 2; prostaglandins were administered in one only.

Uterine rupture occurred in 2 primigravidae. One was due to rupture of the scar of a previous myomectomy at the 16th week, while in the other, rupture was traumatic and associated with delivery by vacuum extraction.

Table 9.2: *Number of women by age who died from the rupture of the uterus in 1976 – 78 compared with 1967 – 75*

Age	1967 – 75			1976 – 78		
	Total maternities	Number of deaths	Rate per million	†Expected deaths on basis of 1967 – 75 rates	Total maternities	Number of actual deaths
Under 25	3,030,081	6	2.0	1	709,038	1
25 – 29	2,161,981	7	3.2	2	637,683	4
30 – 34	967,641	10	10.3	3	303,575	6
35 – 39	402,193	15	37.3	3	79,622	2
40 +	115,315	5	43.4	1	18,931	1
All ages	6,677,211	43	Total (by addition)	10	1,748,849	14

† For method of calculation see page 8

Table 9.3: *Number of women who died from the rupture of the uterus by parity* in 1976 – 78 compared with 1967 – 75*

Parity	1967 – 75			1976 – 78		
	Total maternities	Number of deaths	Rate per million	†Expected deaths on basis of 1967 – 75 rates	Total maternities	Number of actual deaths
1	2,680,166	5	1.9	1	747,409	1
2	2,230,024	7	3.1	2	643,922	4
3	998,707	10	10.0	2	233,388	4
4	417,750	5	12.0	1	76,247	2
5 +	350,564	16	45.6	2	47,885	3
Not stated	—	—	—	—	—	—
All	6,677,211	43	Total (by addition)	8	1,748,849	14

* For definition of parity see page 8
† For method of calculation see page 8

Summary and conclusions

1. Fourteen women died from ruptured uterus.

2. This is 3 more than in 1973 – 75. One death occurred at 16 weeks following rupture of a previous myomectomy scar and 2 other ruptures occurred spontaneously without explanation, at 16 and 29 weeks. Although the triennial incidence has increased for the first time since 1961 – 63, the data must be interpreted with caution when such small numbers are involved.

3. One or more avoidable factors were considered to be present in 11 of the 14 cases.

4. Attention is again drawn to the use of oxytocic drugs in relation to rupture of the uterus, particularly in multiparae and if there as been a previous Caesarean section.

5. Failure to examine the uterine cavity and delay in performing laparotomy when bleeding or shock arise suspicions of rupture of the uterus, are important avoidable factors. Continuing postpartum haemorrhage in the presence of a contracted uterus should cause suspicion of cervical or uterine tears or other damage to the genital tract. There should be no delay in examination and treatment.

6. Each obstetric unit should have an agreed procedure for the treatment of catastrophic haemorrhage, as recommended in Chapters 3 and 8.

10. Amniotic fluid embolism

In this report as in that of 1973 – 75, the diagnosis of death from amniotic fluid embolism has been accepted only when histological examination of lung sections obtained at autopsy provided positive confirmation. In this triennium, 1976 – 78, there were 11 confirmed deaths from amniotic fluid embolism classified under ICD 673.1. The number of deaths in each of the years was 5, 3 and 3 and the death rate per million maternities was 6.3.

Diagnosis

In reports up to 1972, a presumptive clinical diagnosis of amniotic fluid embolism was considered justified by events such as the following:

1. A patient collapsing suddenly, usually after rupture of the membranes. Collapse occurring during labour or within a few hours of delivery. Violent uterine contractions during labour.
2. Collapse accompanied by a fit or muscular twitching and usually with dyspnoea and cyanosis, sometimes with bloodstained frothy mucus coming from the air passages. Intrauterine death of the fetus is not uncommon.
3. Blood coagulation defect, which may be associated with postpartum haemorrhage, continued bleeding after death, or occasionally intra- or retroperitoneal bleeding.

When the 1973 – 75 report was prepared, authoritative pathological opinion indicated that amniotic fluid embolism of a degree sufficient to cause death should be detectable by examination of lung sections stained only by haematoxylin and eosin, although as described in the 1964 – 66 report special stains could make the amniotic squamous cells easier to identify.

It was therefore decided that the diagnosis of amniotic fluid embolism could not be accepted without histological proof and this policy has been continued in the present report. It places a special responsibility on the pathologist at autopsy to take adequate material for full histological examination.

Comparison with previous reports suggests a reduction in the number of deaths in 1976 – 78 (Table 10.1) but with a condition as rare as amniotic embolism, small numbers must be interpreted with caution. These confirmed cases represent a minimal estimate of the number of deaths from amniotic fluid embolism and those cases where amniotic fluid embolism was suspected but not confirmed or not looked for have been included for comparison with the other triennia.

Table 10.1: *Deaths from amniotic fluid embolism, histologically confirmed, and deaths suspected of being amniotic fluid embolism but not confirmed, 1961 – 1978.*

Triennium	1961 – 63	1964 – 66	1967 – 69	1970 – 72	1973 – 75	1976 – 78
Histologically confirmed cases	13	23	20	16	15	11
Suspected cases	14	7	7	8	7	8

All deaths occurred late in pregnancy, the earliest being 31 weeks gestation. All the pregnancies were singletons and of the 11 potentially viable infants, 3 were stillborn (2 delivered by postmortem Caesarean section), 3 died with their undelivered mothers, and one was born alive but died at once, a total of 7 perinatal deaths. Of the 4 surviving infants, one died 6 weeks later, a 'sudden infant death'. Of the 8 women whose infants were actually delivered one was delivered spontaneously, one by forceps, one by vacuum extraction and 5 by Caesarean section, including one 'classical' and 2 'post-mortem' operations.

The first signs of embolism occurred before established labour in 4 cases, in the first stage in 5, in the second stage in one and after delivery in one. Death from embolism occurred before established labour in 2 cases, in the first stage in 4 and after delivery in 5.

Of the 4 who first developed signs before established labour, 2 were delivered by Caesarean section. One was performed as an emergency because of antepartum haemorrhage from placenta praevia. This patient had severe rhesus immunization and had had two previous Caesarean sections. Classical Caesarean section was required because of dense adhesions. Immediately after operation, the patient developed increasing tachycardia and cyanosis and died soon afterwards. The other patient was delivered by Caesarean section because of severe pre-eclampsia at 31 weeks. Initial recovery appeared satisfactory but within 24 hours she developed fever, breathlessness, cyanosis and oliguria. Worsening of her condition necessitated transfer to intensive care but despite artificial ventilation she died 7 days later. The clinical diagnosis was of severe respiratory infection but a very detailed autopsy report revealed typical appearances of amniotic fluid embolism. The two other cases who both developed signs before established labour, suffered placental abruption. Treatment included intravenous oxytocin so that uterine contractions may have been present. Signs of severe concealed placental abruption developed in one patient at rest in hospital at term, with spontaneous rupture of the membranes as well as intrauterine fetal death. During rapid infusion of 2 units of blood she developed a coagulation disorder with bleeding from the gums and extensive skin petechiae and then collapsed and died. In the other patient the presenting sign was slight painless antepartum haemorrhage at term. Examination under anaesthesia excluded placenta praevia and an attempt was made to induce labour by low amniotomy and intravenous oxytocin infusion. The patient collapsed immediately after the procedure and remained cyanosed. A chest radiograph revealed appearances of pulmonary oedema and she died undelivered.

These 4 patients and the 7 patients who had died during labour or after delivery had been admitted to hospital before the amniotic fluid embolism occurred. Of the latter 7 patients, 3 had been admitted because of hypertension, 2 because of spontaneous rupture of the membranes, one because of lower abdominal tenderness at term and previous hysterotomy, and one with polyhydramnios and prolonged pregnancy. The amniotic fluid was later noted to be meconium stained in 4 of these 7 patients but not in any of the 4 women who died before labour was established.

Previous reports have stressed the association of powerful uterine contractions and rapid labour with amniotic fluid embolism. In this series, oxytocic drugs were used in 5 of the 11 cases. In 4, labour was induced, by intravenous oxytocin in 2 and prostaglandin administration in 2, one intravenously and one of the vaginal route. In the remaining patient, intravenous oxytocin was used to accelerate labour because of slow progress after spontaneous rupture of the membranes. Although uterine contractions were noted to be violent in 2 cases, no exceptionally rapid labour was reported. In this series the association with rapid delivery is less obvious than in some previous reports, with 4 deaths occurring before established labour and 5 in first stage labour.

Among the 11 cases there were 5 associated with a coagulation disorder, of whom 4 suffered a postpartum haemorrhage. The other presented with antepartum haemorrhage due to placental abruption, she developed a coagulation disorder and died undelivered.

The last report noted a surprisingly high incidence of abnormalities of the cardiovascular system at autopsy in deaths from amniotic fluid embolism. By contrast in this report, abnormality was found in only one case. This patient collapsed and died 2 hours after the spontaneous onset of labour. Post-mortem Caesarean section was performed but the child died a few minutes after birth. Autopsy confirmed amniotic fluid embolism and also demonstrated a distorted ventricular septum with a large band running obliquely across it.

An avoidable factor was considered to have been present in one case, in which a 'Syntocinon' infusion had been used to stimulate uterine contractions, and this resulted in hypertonic contractions continuing long after the infusion was stopped.

Age and parity

Tables 10.2 and 10.3 show, for histologically confirmed cases, higher rates of mortality at older ages and higher parity. Over the period 1970 – 78 for those aged 35 years and over the rate was 41.2 per million maternities compared with 4.7 for those under 35 years. For women of parity 4 and over the mortality rate was 29.1 per million maternities compared with 4.8 for those of para 1 to 3. (The distribution by age and parity for histologically confirmed cases was not available before 1970).

Some of the older highly parous women had social and family problems and the present pregnancy occurred some years after the previous one. For example, in the 8 multiparous women aged 30 years or more, the time interval from the previous to this pregnancy was 11 years in 2 women, 8, 9 and 13 years respectively in 3 women and in only 3 was the interval as short as 2 or 3 years.

Table 10.2: *Number of women by age who died from histologically confirmed amniotic fluid embolism in 1976 – 78 compared with 1970 – 75*

| | 1970 – 75 | | | | 1976 – 78 | |
Age	Total maternities	Number of deaths	Rate per million	†Expected deaths on basis of 1970 – 75 rates	Total maternities	Number of actual deaths
Under 25	1,900,262	10	5.3	4	709,038	1
25 – 29	1,438,064	6	4.2	3	637,683	1
30 – 34	591,309	2	3.4	1	303,575	6
35 – 39	227,045	7	30.8	2	79,622	3
40 +	63,087	6	95.1	2	18,931	–
All ages	4,219,767	31	Total by addition	12	1,748,849	11

Table 10.3: *Number of women by parity* who died from histologically confirmed amniotic fluid embolism in 1976 – 78 compared with 1970 – 75*

| | 1970 – 75 | | | | 1976 – 78 | |
Parity	Total maternities	Number of deaths	Rate per million	†Expected deaths on basis of 1970 – 75 rates	Total maternities	Number of actual deaths
1	1,733,916	7	4.0	3	747,409	3
2	1,451,789	8	5.5	4	643,922	3
3	609,205	2	3.3	1	233,388	3
4	241,338	5	20.7	2	76,247	1
5 +	183,519	9	49.0	2	47,885	1
All	4,219,767	31	Total by addition	12	1,748,849	11

* For definition of parity see page 8
† For method of calculation see page 8

Comments

The number of histologically proven cases of amniotic fluid embolism in this report (11) is 4 less than in the last report and may represent a decrease in incidence. The birthrate reached its lowest level in 1977 however and although it began to rise in 1978, the decrease in incidence is not significant. Since there has been no improvement in the detection or management of amniotic fluid embolism, a decrease might be related to either a reduction in the proportion of older or higher multiparous women in the pregnant population.

Although oxytocic drugs were used in 5 of the 11 cases however, the relationship between violent contractions and rapid labour is less apparent in this report than in previous reports.

Summary and conclusions

1. In this report there were 11 histologically proved deaths from amniotic fluid embolism.

2. Three women died undelivered, and 2 were delivered by post-mortem Caesarean section. Of the 11 potentially viable infants, 7 died in the perinatal period, a mortality rate of 64%.

3. Violent uterine action was noted in only one case and progress at labour was not judged to be unduly precipitate in any of the 11 deaths. Oxytocic drugs were used in 5 cases, oxytocin in 3 and prostaglandin in 2. The fact that uterine hyperactivity was reported in only one case in this report may reflect a more cautious use of oxytocic drugs in general. The administration of oxytocic drugs should be controlled with the greatest care, particularly in multiparous and older women, in whom sudden acceleration of labour can occur with dramatic swiftness despite previous slow progress.

4. Coagulation failure occurred in 5 patients and was associated with postpartum haemorrhage in 4 cases.

5. Avoidable factors were considered to have been present in one case in whom unduly strong uterine contractions appeared to develop after administration of oxytocic drugs.

6. Abnormalities of the maternal cardiovascular system were noted at autopsy in only one of 11 cases, in contrast with 6 of 15 cases in the previous report.

7. Amniotic fluid embolism remains an unpredictable and largely unpreventable cause of maternal death. Inclusion of histologically confirmed cases only will at least prevent the too easy designation of death to amniotic fluid embolism and help to ensure that other possible causes including gram-negative septicaemia are searched for when proof of amniotic fluid embolism is not found. A special onus is placed on pathologists to take adequate material at autopsy for histological analysis.

11. Ectopic pregnancy

Twenty one maternal deaths directly caused by ectopic pregnancy occurred during the years 1976, 1977 and 1978; the number for each of these years was 7, 9 and 5 respectively. In 18 instances the pregnancy was in the Fallopian tube (ICD 633.1) in 2 cases there was a primary ovarian pregnancy (ICD 633.2), and one cornual pregnancy (ICD 633.8).

As uterine haemorrhage, abortion, hypertensive diseases of pregnancy, pulmonary embolism and sepsis become relatively less common other complications of pregnancy and childbirth play a greater part and failure to anticipate, diagnose or treat them successfully becomes more significant. This is certainly so with ectopic pregnancy in which the great hazard is difficulty with diagnosis. Later in this chapter details will be given of a woman developing gastro-intestinal symptoms in the evening and being found dead next morning; of a woman with simultaneous intra- and extra-uterine pregnancies both progressing nearly to term, and of a death from ectopic pregnancy in a woman who had had a bilateral tubal ligation.

Another patient died of faecal peritonitis after a difficult laparotomy by a junior member of the gynaecological staff. This case has been included in Chapter 12.

One death associated with ectopic pregnancy occurred from an anaesthetic mishap and this case has been included in the chapter of deaths associated with anaesthesia rather than as an ectopic pregnancy death and has been included in Chapter 8 and coded to ICD 668.

Comparison of the number of women who died from ectopic pregnancy in the triennia since 1952 and about whom the MCW 97 forms were completed and the corresponding Registrar General's figures are shown in Table 11.1. It will be noted that in this triennium all known cases of death from ectopic pregnancy were reported indicating the completeness of the Enquiry. This should be contrasted with the discrepancies due to failure of reporting in the earlier years.

Table 11.1: *The number of women who died from ectopic pregnancy 1952 – 78*

Triennia	1952–1954	1955–1957	1958–1960	1961–1963	1964–1966	1967–1969	1970–1972	1973–1975	1976–1978
Maternal deaths from ectopic pregnancy	59	42	28	42	42	32	34	21	21
Registrar General's figures	78	62	42	50	49	39	36	22	21

Table 11.2: Deaths from ectopic pregnancy and rates per million estimated conceptions 1970 – 72, 1973 – 75 and 1976 – 78

Year	All abortions in HIPE	Ectopic pregnancies in HIPE	Non-NHS Legal abortions	Maternities	Total estimated conceptions	Ectopic pregnancies per 1,000,000 estimated conceptions	Ectopic deaths	Death rate per million estimated conceptions
1970 – 72	366,100	11,620	121,411	2,298,201	2,797,332	420	34	12.2
1973 – 75	338,430	11,710	163,764	1,921,568	2,430,472	480	21	8.6
1976 – 78	317,090	11,580	158,301	1,748,851	2,235,822	520	21	9.4

The fact of pregnancy is not legally notifiable until the 28th week of pregnancy after which registration of a live or stillbirth becomes a statutory obligation. Therefore there is some difficulty in estimating the number of women at risk from ectopic pregnancy. However the number of deaths from ectopic pregnancy has been compared with the number of conceptions, estimated by the method described in Chapter 1 (see Table 11.2).

Table 11.2 shows that there was little difference in the death rate per million estimated conceptions between 1973 – 75 and 1976 – 78, despite the fact that the proportion of conceptions with an outcome of ectopic pregnancy has steadily risen since 1970.

Duration of amenorrhoea

During 1976 – 78 this varied between 6 and 37 weeks at the time of death as follows:—

Duration of amenorrhoea	*Number of cases*
< 7 weeks	7
7 – 8 weeks	3
9 – 10 weeks	1
16 weeks	1
37 weeks	1
Not stated	8

Table 11.3: *Duration of amenorrhoea at the time of death from ectopic pregnancy 1970 – 78*

Duration of amenorrhoea in weeks	Number of cases			Total 1970 – 78
	1970 – 72	1973 – 75	1976 – 78	
< 7 weeks	13	4	7	24
7 – 8 weeks	7	7	3	17
9 – 10 weeks	3	2	1	6
11 – 12 weeks	4	1	–	5
13 – 14 weeks	2	1	–	3
15 – 16 weeks	1	1	1	3
17 – 18 weeks	1	–	–	1
19 – 20 weeks	–	1	–	1
21 – 22 weeks	–	1	–	1
23 – 24 weeks	1	–	–	1
37 weeks	–	–	1	1
Not stated	2	3	8	13
Total	34	21	21	76

Racial status

In previous reports comments have been made about the apparent relatively greater proportion of women dying of an ectopic pregnancy who were of non-Caucasian origin. This relationship is not apparent in the years covered by the present report as only two women were non-caucasian. The figures since 1964 were as follows:—

Years	Non-Caucasian women dying from ectopic pregnancy expressed as a percentage of all women dying from ectopic pregnancy
1964 – 66	30%
1967 – 69	38%
1970 – 72	32%
1973 – 75	43%
1976 – 78	10%

Clinical features and avoidable factors

One or more avoidable factors were present in 6 of the 21 deaths. In one instance a single woman aged 18 denied the possibility of pregnancy. She consulted her general practitioner who did not examine her although she complained of faintness, abdominal pain, diarrhoea and vomiting. She collapsed at work on the same day and was dead on arrival at hospital.

There were 2 cases of women being admitted for investigation of suspected spontaneous abortion and having a dilatation and curettage of the uterus. In one instance the uterine contents were not sent for a histological examination. These patients died 7 and 9 days respectively after discharge from hospital. One was awaiting a laparoscopic examination and the other admission for sterilization.

One patient was admitted to a gynaecological ward and there was delay in the line of communication between the house surgeon, registrar and consultant and delay before laparotomy. 'Large amounts of blood and clot' were found in the peritoneal cavity and the woman died from cardiac arrest in the operating theatre.

Two women were admitted to the care of general surgeons. In both cases there was evidence of over-transfusion post-operatively. One woman lost 400 ml and was transfused with 3,000 ml of blood and other fluids and developed pulmonary oedema. In the other there was a 3 hour delay in opening the abdomen. She had a blood loss of 900 ml. In the first 36 hours after operation she was transfused with 9,500 ml of blood. She died of pulmonary oedema and cardiac failure. Seven of the 14 patients in whom no avoidable factors were identified died suddenly at home or were dead or moribund on arrival at hospital.

One patient was admitted to a medical ward in a diabetic coma and the coincident ectopic pregnancy was not recognized. No avoidable factor was considered to be present in this case.

One woman died of ectopic pregnancy despite oral contraception with a combined oestrogen and progestogen preparation.

In one death the woman had had salpingostomy and salpingolysis for infertility, and in another the woman had been sterilized.

In no case was an intra-uterine contraceptive device being used or found at autopsy.

Of special interest is the case where the pregnancy proceeded to the 37th week of gestation. When she was admitted to the antenatal ward at the 28th week because of faintness and lower abdominal pain radiological examination revealed the presence of twins. She was readmitted in the 37th week of pregnancy in severe shock. No fetal heart was heard; the cervix was effaced and the membranes were bulging without any vaginal bleeding. She died half an hour after admission. At post-mortem examination there was found a near term twin pregnancy with one fetus in the uterine cavity and another in the left ovary, the ovarian tissue over the placenta had torn with subsequent haemorrhage into the abdominal cavity.

One unmarried woman (who did not know she was pregnant) had been treated by her general practitioner for a complaint of diarrhoea and vomiting. She was seen by her general practitioner the evening before she was found dead in bed.

The number of women in the enquiry series, who died from ectopic pregnancy analysed by age and parity from 1970–78 is shown in Tables 11.4 and 11.5. The total estimated death rate per million conceptions, and that for each triennium are also shown in Table 11.4.

Table 11.4: *Number of women in the enquiry series, who died from ectopic pregnancy, by age, 1970–78, and estimated death rate per million conceptions for each triennium*

Age (years)	Number of deaths			
	1970–72	1973–75	1976–78	Total
16–19	2	4	1	7
20–24	5	1	3	9
25–29	7	5	5	17
30–34	11	4	2	17
35–39	7	5	6	18
40–44	2	2	4	8
16–44	34	21	21	76
Estimated death rate per million conceptions	12.2	8.6	9.4	10.2

Table 11.5: *Number of women in the enquiry series, who died from ectopic pregnancy by parity*, 1970 – 78*

Parity*	Number of deaths			
	1970 – 72	1973 – 75	1976 – 78	Total
1	12	10	11	33
2	9	–	1	10
3	7	4	3	14
4	1	3	2	6
5+	3	2	4	9
Not stated	2	2	–	4
All	34	21	21	76

* For definition of parity see page 8

Summary and conclusions

1. During the triennium the mortality from ectopic pregnancy was one third of that recorded in the first report 1952 – 1954 and one half of that recorded for the years 1964 – 66 when a chapter on ectopic pregnancy was first included. However since 1970 the mortality rate has not improved, and may be worsening.

2. Avoidable factors, single or multiple were present in 6 deaths, due to failure to investigate fully or to errors in the management of bleeding. In two instances over-transfusion contributed to the deaths.

3. In 7 instances the women collapsed so suddenly that there was no chance of treatment.

4. There was no evidence during 1976 – 78 that a woman of non-Caucasian racial origin has a greater likelihood of dying from an ectopic pregnancy than a Caucasian woman in contrast with findings of the previous 4 reports.

5. The proportion of conceptions with an ectopic outcome has apparently risen since 1970 but there was little difference in the death rate per million estimated conceptions between 1976 – 78 and 1973 – 75.

6. No woman was found to have an intra-uterine device *in situ*; one woman was taking a combined oral contraceptive pill.

7. Two women had had previous tubal surgery, one for infertility and one for sterilization.

12.   Puerperal sepsis

There were 24 deaths due to infection of the genital tract in 1976, 1977 and 1978. They have been classified as follows:

Sepsis after abortion	ICD 634 – 637	7
Major puerperal infection	ICD 670	8
Sepsis after surgical	⎰ ICD 639.2	1
procedures	⎱ ICD 670	8

Deaths from sepsis after abortion are also considered in Chapter 5 and those connected with Caesarean section are also considered in Chapter 7. Two deaths occurred more than 42 days after abortion or delivery and would be excluded under the international* definition of maternal death. No other deaths from sepsis are known to have occurred.

Comparison with the triennial report 1970 – 72 shows that the reduction in the number of deaths or the death rates from abortion with sepsis, puerperal sepsis or sepsis after surgical procedures in 1973 – 75 has been maintained. (See Table 12.1)

Table 12.1: *Maternal deaths from sepsis, with estimated rates per million maternities, 1952 – 78*

	1952 – 54	1955 – 57	1958 – 60	1961 – 63	1964 – 66	1967 – 69	1970 – 72	1973 – 75	1976 – 78
Sepsis after abortion	91	82	77	74	66	62	38	6	7
Puerperal sepsis	42	46	24	18	28	12	15	11	8
Sepsis after surgical procedures	26	30	23	19	29	14	17	11	9
Total	159	158	124	111	123	88	70	28	24
Rates per million maternities	77.4	74.8	54.0	44.0	47.3	35.8	30.5	14.6	13.7

As in previous reports, infections not involving the genital tract are included in other chapters.

Sepsis after abortion

There were 7 deaths from sepsis after abortion, 3 followed illegal abortion and 4 legal abortion.

* see page 7

One other patient aborted spontaneously and died from disseminated intra-vascular coagulation and haemolytic streptococcal septicaemia and has been included in Chapter 14 as varicella was the primary infection.

Illegal abortion

One woman concealed her abortion and was admitted to hospital moribund with a haemoglobin concentration of 1.5 g/dl, after bleeding continuously for 2 weeks. The uterus contained adherent and infected placenta. In the second case, a self-induced abortion occurred in the woman's home and was followed by infection of retained placental tissue. She died 2 weeks later from septicaemia due to *E Coli* and *β- haemolytic streptococci*, cultured also from the uterus. Autopsy revealed micro-abscesses in various organs. The third patient was found dead and autopsy revealed death to be due to *Cl. welchii* septicaemia from uterine infection due to abortion induced by soap solution.

Legal abortion

Of the 4 deaths following legal abortion, 2 were due to septicaemia associated with *Cl. welchii* infection. In the first case, extra-amniotic administration of prostaglandins was used to induce abortion. The placenta was retained and at manual removal under anaesthesia the patient was noted to be febrile and ampicillin was administered. Jaundice, cyanosis and hypotension quickly developed and she died within 6 hours. The second patient was allowed home on the day after a vaginal termination of pregnancy performed under general anaesthesia at the 10th week. She developed abdominal pain on the day after discharge and was treated conservatively by her general practitioner. She collapsed and died, and autopsy revealed a *Cl. welchii* septicaemia, pelvic peritonitis and a whole fetus within the uterus.

The 2 other deaths were associated with peritonitis. One was caused by rupture of the uterus during vaginal termination performed by a registrar. The consultant confirmed the uterine rupture, and carried out total abdominal hysterectomy. She developed paralytic ileus and died on the 10th post-operative day. Autopsy revealed generalized peritonitis with the bowel loops matted together consistent with a diagnosis of previous perforation of the small intestine. In the other case, an obese hypertensive woman who had had 2 previous Caesarean sections, a termination of pregnancy was attempted by extra-amniotic and, later, vaginal administration of prostaglandins, as well as with intravenous oxytocin. When abortion had not occurred after 7 days, examination under anaesthesia revealed uterine rupture. Laparotomy confirmed this diagnosis, the rupture being fundal and not through the previous lower segment scars. The rupture was repaired and the patient died 5 days later of bacteraemic shock associated with generalized peritonitis.

Avoidable factors were considered to be present in 6 of the 7 cases. As in previous reports an avoidable factor was attributed to the patient in all 3 cases of illegal abortion and in one of these also to the general practitioner, whose management predisposed to delay in the provision of effective treatment. In 3 of the 4 cases of legal abortion an avoidable factor was attributed to the consultant team, and in one of these also to the general practitioner.

Major puerperal infection

This category excludes women who died after Caesarean section and other surgical procedures. Eight maternal deaths were caused by puerperal sepsis and of these 6 had spontaneous rupture of the membranes in labour, one had artificial rupture of the membranes at term and in another case the membranes were ruptured in labour. No labour was known to be prolonged more than 24 hours.

Two women were delivered without medical or nursing attention. One woman failed to keep any antenatal or booking appointments. The couple would not admit the diagnosis of advanced pregnancy even when they were about to be married, but 5 days later a mature 3.9 kg infant was delivered in the holiday caravan in which they were spending their honeymoon. The infant died almost at once and autopsy later revealed hemicrania, the skull containing only clear fluid. Two days after delivery, the patient became ill, developed diarrhoea and travelled to hospital by public transport. *Haemolytic streptococci* were cultured from vaginal swabs and blood samples and the patient died 20 days after delivery from respiratory and hepato-renal failure. Another couple agreed to keep pregnancy and labour secret. A stillborn child was delivered without medical or nursing attention. The mother died 3 days postpartum, still without qualified care. Autopsy revealed the uterus still enlarged to 20 weeks pregnancy size with florid endometritis. *Haemolytic* streptococci were cultured from the uterus and lungs confirming a diagnosis of septicaemia.

Of the 8 women who died from puerperal sepsis, 5 had spontaneous deliveries, 2 had forceps deliveries and in one woman with twins the first twin was delivered spontaneously and the second by forceps. In her case, rapidly progressive *Cl. sordelli* infection developed in the pelvis and perineum, spread to the buttocks, abdominal wall and lateral pelvic walls and she died on the 7th day. The second twin delivered by forceps, died of the same infection, spreading from the umbilicus.

One other woman delivered by forceps discharged herself against medical advice 48 hours after delivery, despite abdominal pain and difficulty with micturition. She was readmitted 3 days later with acute retention of urine and septicaemia, *Proteus mirabilis* being cultured from the vagina, urine and blood. Despite appropriate antibiotic therapy, she died 10 days later of respiratory and renal failure. Autopsy revealing an infected uterus and gross bilateral pyelonephritis with abscess formation.

In the third woman, following delivery by forceps, an extensive vaginal tear was found and apparently repaired satisfactorily by a senior house officer. Postnatal examination was not arranged. The patient was depressed and was admitted to a mental hosptial about 8 months later, suffering also from weight loss, diarrhoea and faecal incontinence. A recto-vaginal fistula was ultimately detected but the patient was moribund by the time she was transferred to a surgical unit. At autopsy, a recto-vaginal fistula 1 cm in diameter was found with an adjacent labyrinth of extra peritoneal abscesses and necrosis of both ilio-psoas muscles. This case would be excluded under the international* definition of maternal mortality because she died 10 months after delivery.

One other patient would also be excluded as she died 17 weeks after a normal spontaneous delivery. She was then admitted having been unconscious for 24 hours. Septicaemia was detected and she died 2 days later despite treatment. A mixture of pathogenic organisms was cultured from vaginal swabs. Autopsy revealed a sloughing, infected area in the vaginal vault with infected myometrium and an ulcerated cervix.

This latter case, and the two women who died unattended, represent 3 of the 5 spontaneous deliveries. Of the remaining 2, one was delivered at home as planned, and died 3 days later of rapidly progressing septicaemia arising from an infected episiotomy wound. The other developed jaundice in late pregnancy possibly due to infective hepatitis. Labour was induced, but the infant was stillborn. The mother developed paralytic ileus and subsequently died of *E. coli* septicaemia. Autopsy was not performed.

Avoidable factors were attributed to both patients who delivered unattended and also to the patient who discharged herself against medical advice. Avoidable factors were also attributed to the consultant team in one case.

Sepsis after Surgical Procedures

The 9 deaths under this heading were associated with lower segment Caesarean section in 8 and in one with laparotomy for an ectopic pregnancy.

Three of the deaths from Caesarean section were due to peritonitis from perforation of the bowel. The sites of the perforations were mid-ileum, caecum and transverse colon.

Of the other 5 deaths due to infection following Caesarean section, one followed a coagulation defect due to *B proteus* septicaemia. This patient had been unwilling to come into hospital for investigation of proteinuria and persistent urinary infection due to *B proteus*. The other 4 deaths were all assocated with severe uterine sepsis leading to peritonitis and septicaemia. The organisms involved included *haemolytic streptococci*, pneumococci, *Cl. welchii*, and bacteroides. One of these patients had a cervical cerclage at 16 weeks. She was subsequently delivered by elective Caesarean section because of some antepartum haemorrhage. Following delivery the patient developed pyrexia. Her condition rapidly deteriorated with rigors and septic shock. Despite intensive treatment, she died 9 days after delivery. Autopsy confirmed the presence of septicaemia the organisms being anaerobic streptococci and bacteroides.

The death which occurred following laparotomy for ectopic pregnancy was due to perforation of the sigmoid colon confirmed at autopsy.

Three other deaths should be mentioned here, 2 due to haemorrhage included in Chapter 3 and one to cardiac disease included in Chapter 6, in which sepsis following a surgical procedure played a significant part. In one,

* See page 7

110

the patient developed *Klebsiella* septicaemia following elective Caesarean section complicated by postpartum haemorrhage with coagulation defect. The septicaemia did not respond to antibiotics and at hysterectomy the uterus was necrotic.

Another patient had a cervical suture removed at 37 weeks of pregnancy. Labour later began spontaneously and in the second stage, the patient collapsed, apparently as a result of amniotic fluid embolism. Forceps delivery was followed by massive postpartum haemorrhage which was never completely controlled until hysterectomy was performed a day later. The uterus was full of micro abscesses. When the patient died some days later, autopsy revealed death to be due to septicaemia, without evidence of amniotic fluid embolism.

The third death followed emergency Caesarean section for prolapsed cord. Four days after discharge, the patient was readmitted seriously ill with septicaemia and recurrent episodes of bacteraemic shock. She died 27 days after delivery of infective endocarditis, due to *E. coli* and *B proteus*.

Avoidable factors were considered to be present in 7 of the 9 cases. The patient alone and the general practitioner alone were each involved in one case and the consultant team alone in 3 cases. In one case, both the consultant team and the patient were involved, and in another case, both the consultant team and the general practitioner were involved.

Summary and conclusions

1. The reduction noted in the previous triennium, 1973 – 75, has been maintained compared with the previous triennia.

2. The marked improvement in the number of deaths associated with sepsis after abortion achieved in 1973 – 75 has been maintained.

3. Avoidable factors were present in 17 of the total of 24 deaths from sepsis. Included in this are 6 of the 7 deaths from sepsis after abortion, 4 of 8 deaths after vaginal delivery, and 7 of 9 deaths after surgical procedures.

4. Sepsis of the genital tract particularly when associated with anaerobic organisms may present in a wide variety of forms even without pyrexia. When associated with collapse or haemorrhage in labour or the puerperium, earlier diagnosis and more effective treatment requires constant awareness of its potential presence. Close collaboration with a microbiologist is essential. If abdominal complications occur, there should be early consultation with a general surgeon and readiness to reopen the abdomen.

5. Attention is drawn to the number of deaths from bowel perforation following obstetrical procedures. There was one death from rupture of the caecum and 3 deaths from perforation of the mid ileum, the transverse colon and the sigmoid colon as well as a late death due to a recto-vaginal fistula.

6. Attention is also drawn to the occurrence of uterine infection and septicaemia in association with the use of cervical cerclage.

13. Deaths from miscellaneous causes

Since the 1964 – 66 report an account has been given of some of the causes of maternal deaths which do not easily fit into the other chapters. In other instances the unusual nature of the cause of death merits comment and there are cases in which no known cause of death could be found.

Twenty cases of death from miscellaneous causes occurred in the years 1976 – 78, and are described in this chapter together with 2 cases coded to abortion and one to haemorrhage.

The 20 cases have been coded by the International Classification of Diseases 9th edition as follows:—

ICD Number	Diagnosis	Number of cases
674.9	Sudden death of unknown cause in puerperium	6
646.9	Sudden death of unknown cause in pregnancy	1
646.7	Liver disorders in pregnancy	7
673.0	Obstetrical air embolism	1
181	Malignant neoplasm of placenta	1
643.2	Excessive vomiting in late pregnancy	1
669.4	Cerebral anoxia following obstetrical surgery	1
669.8	Other complications of delivery (inhalation of gastric contents)	1
671.5	Venous complications of pregnancy and the puerperium	1

Sudden death of unknown cause in peurperium

There were 6 deaths in this group. In 4 instances it was the woman's first pregnancy and in 2 it was the second pregnancy.

Two deaths occurred in hospital one on the day following forceps delivery and one 20 days after Caesarean section. Four women died at home between 22 to 40 days after vaginal delivery in hospital.

In one of the six deaths a full post-mortem examination was performed, but no cause was found. In the other cases it was considered that more careful post-mortem examination might have revealed the cause of death.

Sudden death of unknown cause in pregnancy

There was one woman aged 27 who had a laparotomy at the eleventh week of her second pregnancy, for a suspected ectopic pregnancy. A normal intra-uterine pregnancy was found together with an ovarian cyst which was removed. She was found dead at home 3 weeks later having appeared to be perfectly well. Postmortem examination including histology provided no convincing cause of death.

Liver disorders in pregnancy

There were 7 deaths from liver disorders, 4 being diagnosed as 'fatty liver of pregnancy', one as 'acute hepatic necrosis' and two as 'hepatic failure'.

One West African patient was admitted to hospital with jaundice and vomiting at the 34th week of pregnancy and died 8 days after emergency Caesarean section. Four other cases had jaundice and vomiting between the 32nd and 38th weeks of pregnancy. They were all delivered normally and died a few days afterwards. One woman aged 18 was treated for Still's disease with corticosteroids and died undelivered at the 38th week of gestation with hepatic necrosis.

Air embolism

One woman aged 29 and in her fourth pregnancy was booked for home delivery. At the 44th week of pregnancy labour started spontaneously and within 65 minutes cervical dilatation progressed from 2 to 10 centimetres. The patient pushed twice, had a fit and died undelivered. Postmortem examination showed pulmonary air embolism but no histological examination was made of the lungs.

There were 2 instances of air embolism associated with abortion and avoidable factors were judged to be present in both. A woman aged 20 in her first pregnancy of 7 weeks duration, was found dead at home after an attempted illegal abortion. Bubbles of air were found in the pulmonary arteries. There was no mention in the report about the method used to induce the abortion. A woman aged 37, having her third pregnancy legally aborted at the 18th week by intra-amniotic prostaglandin and urea, had a convulsion and died from air embolism. Two attempts at amniocentesis had been required before amniotic fluid was aspirated and the prostaglandin and urea injected.

Choriocarcinoma

There was one case of an 18 year old primigravida who had a normal pregnancy and labour and was admitted to hospital 12 weeks postpartum with dyspnoea and haemoptysis. She died 10 days later from choriocarcinoma. She would therefore be excluded under the international* definition of maternal death. As in previous reports, the death is discussed here under miscellaneous causes of true maternal death. The ICD does not classify choriocarcinoma as a complication of pregnancy and childbirth, and for statistical purposes, deaths are coded as 'associated' with pregnancy (ICD 181).

It is worthy of note that 8 patients with choriocarcinoma died during 1976 – 78 who are not recorded in this report because they all died more than a year after pregnancy, 3 of these being from abroad and receiving treatment for the disease in this country.

Excessive vomiting in late pregnancy

This woman was aged 31 and started vomiting at the 28th week of her second pregnancy. She inhaled vomit and died of pneumonia.

Inhalation of gastric contents

A woman collapsed in labour at term and inhaled gastric contents. A post-mortem Caesarean section (included in Chapter 7 Addendum) resulted in the delivery of a stillborn fetus. Avoidable factors were attributed to the consultant team.

Retroperitoneal haematoma

This case is included in Chapter 3. A 32 year old woman pregnant for the 5th time, had a spontaneous delivery complicated by antepartum and postpartum haemorrhages and by disseminated intravascular coagulation. At laparotomy to control bleeding the small bowel was found to be severely infarcted by a large retroperioneal haematoma.

Cerebral sinus thrombosis

A 42 year old Indian woman of unknown parity was admitted to hospital with grand mal fits about the 10th week of pregnancy. She died 3 days later. Autopsy revealed pelvic vein and cerebral sinus thrombosis.

* see page 7

14.   Associated causes of maternal deaths

There were 200 deaths from diseases associated with but not directly due to obstetric complications of which 21 were the deaths from cardiac disease which have been included in Chapter 6.

As described in Chapter I these have been divided into *indirect* maternal deaths or *fortuitous* deaths. Ninety-seven deaths were classified as indirect and 103 as fortuitous.

Indirect maternal deaths are defined as those resulting from a previously existing disease, or disease that developed during pregnancy and which did not have a direct obstetric cause but which was aggravated by the physiological effects of pregnancy. This definition has also been interpreted here to cover deaths where the presence of the existing disease and the pregnancy were inter-related and the disease resulted in significant changes in the treatment or management of the pregnancy.

Fortuitous deaths have been classified as those in which women were known to have been pregnant at the time of death or within one year of death, but which were apparently either not related to the pregnancy or not aggravated by it, such as death from a road traffic accident. Nineteen of the indirect deaths occurred more than 42 days after delivery and would be excluded under the international* definition of maternal death, as would all the fortuitous deaths. Forty-seven of the fortuitous deaths also occurred more than 42 days after delivery. The fortuitous deaths have all been marked (†) in this chapter.

Adrenal Disorders

There were two patients who died as a result of adrenal hypofunction and both were considered to be indirect deaths.

One patient, a primigravida aged 38 years had had a bilateral adrenalectomy for congenital adrenal hyperplasia, and was maintained on steroid therapy. She was well until 24 weeks of pregnancy when she developed an adrenal crisis. She was admitted to hospital but died the same day.

The other patient had a spontaneous delivery at 35 weeks gestation after an uneventful pregnancy. She was found dead at home 7 months postpartum having had a two day history of sore throat, weakness, nausea and vomiting. At the post-mortem examination she was found to have acute pericarditis and adrenal hypoplasia.

* See page 7

Arterial aneurysms

There were 5 deaths as the result of the rupture of arterial aneurysms, all classified as indirect deaths. There was one death from rupture of an aneurysm of the hepatic artery. The patient was admitted at 32 weeks gestation with abdominal pain and strong uterine contractions and was allowed to go home the same day because nothing abnormal was found. She returned a few hours later complaining of pain in her back and abdomen. She was treated with analgesics and died 4 hours later. Two patients died from rupture of a dissecting aneurysm of the aorta. One died 10 days following a normal delivery and the other was found dead at home in her 36th week of pregnancy. No evidence of Marfan's syndrome was found by the pathologist in either case.

The 4th patient, para 2, aged 32 years was well until the 34th week of pregnancy. She was then admitted to hospital with severe chest pain and was treated with herapin for pulmonary embolism. She died a few hours later and was found at autopsy to have had a rupture of an aneurysm of the splenic artery.

The 5th patient was admitted with severe epigastric pain at 30 weeks gestation in her second pregnancy. She was thought to have had a placental abruption when she became pale and shocked 3 hours after admission. She died from haemorrhage associated with abnormal left renal arteries. An avoidable factor was attributed to the obstetric team because the consultant had not been informed of the patient's admission.

Alcoholic disorders

One patient, whose death was considered to be indirect, was formerly an alcoholic and had cirrhosis of the liver. She declined an offer of termination of pregnancy. She was admitted as an emergency and died the same day of haemorrhage from oesophageal varices at the 23rd week of gestation.

There was one fortuitous† death when a patient died from a vasovagal attack caused by excessive and probably rapid intake of alcohol two months after delivery.

Auto-immune diseases

One patient aged 32 years with systemic sclerosis died 14 weeks after her third delivery. She had been under treatment for 5 years and during her pregnancy the condition had been in remission. Following delivery the sclerosis worsened and despite intensive treatment she died from bronchopneumonia. This was considered to be an indirect death but would be excluded under the international* definition of maternal death. Another patient died from systemic lupus erythematosus when about 28 weeks into her first pregnancy. She was known to have lupoid hepatitis for which she was receiving cortico-

* See page 7

116

steroids. Termination of pregnancy had been considered but it had been decided that it would probably be safe to let it continue. At 20 weeks gestation she had a haemorrhage from oesophageal varices. She died after further haemorrhages and at post-mortem examination the fetus was found to be macerated in utero. This case was classified as an indirect death.

Blood diseases

There were 10 deaths, either caused by blood diseases, or to which these contributed:

i. *Sickle cell disease* One patient from East Africa died following a lower segment Caesarean section for fetal distress. She was known to have sickle cell trait and also glucose-6-phosphate dehydrogenase deficiency. She had a cardiac arrest about 2 hours after the operation, having appeared to be making a satisfactory recovery. Despite resuscitation she died the same day from haemorrhage and the sickle cell trait was judged to have been a contributory factor. The case is included in Chapter 3.

The three other cases of sickle cell disease were regarded as indirect deaths. In the first a West Indian primigravida was under investigation for homozygous sickle cell disease. Three days before her death, at 20 weeks gestation she complained of back pains which were considered by her general practitioner to be caused by a urinary infection. Two days later she had a severe epistaxis and was admitted to hospital. Her haemoglobin on admission was 1.7 g/dl and she was found to be in congestive cardiac failure. Death was attributed to disseminated intravascular coagulation due to acute haemolysis.

A nineteen year old primigravida from Saudi Arabia was in the United Kingdom on holiday. She was between 4 and 5 months pregnant. She complained of pain in her legs and back which was associated with pyrexia and a diagnosis of a viral infection was made. The following day she was admitted to hospital deeply unconscious and died soon after admission. Post-mortem examination showed that her death was due to a sickle cell crisis.

The third patient was a primigravida aged 18 years from Guyana. She had a long history of psychiatric disorder and was judged to be unable to cope with her pregnancy. At 20 weeks gestation, it was decided to terminate the pregnancy with intra-amniotic injection of prostaglandin and urea. She collapsed 30 minutes after the amniocentesis, and death was due to a sickle cell cris. The haemoglobinopathy not having been detected prior to the procedure.

ii. *Acute leukaemia* Four women died from acute leukaemia.

There were 3 deaths from myeloid leukaemia which were classified as indirect maternal deaths. The first patient, a primigravida aged 19 years, was well until 34 weeks gestation when acute myeloid leukaemia was diagnosed. Labour was induced 2 weeks later. Despite chemotherapy she died 41 days postpartum.

A 17 year old primigravida from Pakistan was first found to be anaemic at 22 weeks of pregnancy. The anaemia failed to respond to treatment and acute myeloid leukaemia was diagnosed 10 weeks later. She had a premature delivery and collapsed and died 36 hours later with severe abdominal pain and shock. Permission for a post-mortem examination was refused but she was thought to have died from an intra-abdominal haemorrhage. The third patient was transferred from Kuwait after the diagnosis of myeloid leukaemia had been made at 28 weeks gestation, and chemotherapy treatment begun. She died six hours after the premature delivery of a macerated stillborn fetus.

One death from lymphatic leukaemia, occurring 11 months after a normal pregnancy and delivery, was regarded as fortuitous†.

iii. *Thrombocytopenic purpura* There was one death from thrombocytopenic purpura which was considered to be a fortuitous† death.

iv. *Thrombotic thrombocytropenic purpura* in pregnancy. There was one death from this condition which was classified as an indirect maternal death. The patient aged 21 years had a history of haemolytic anaemia associated with her previous pregnancy. Following an emergency Caesarean section for fetal distress at 36 weeks of pregnancy, her haemoglobin was 6.6 g/dl and platelets 33,000/cu mm. She was treated with corticosteroids and repeated blood transfusions. Twelve days after delivery hemiplegia developed which was shown to have been caused by an infarction. Despite appropriate treatment she died suddenly two months after delivery. Post-mortem examination revealed extensive intrapulmonary haemorrhage and petechial haemorrhages in all organs of the body. This case would be excluded under the international* definition of maternal death.

Cerebral infarction

There were three deaths from cerebral infarction.

Two of these were considered to be indirect. A woman, para 2, aged 27 years, had been induced at 41 weeks and was delivered by forceps. Quinestrol was given to suppress lactation. Four days after delivery she developed hemiplegia and became comatose and died 8 days after delivery. Autopsy revealed a thrombosis of the left internal carotoid artery with massive infarction of the left cerebral hemisphere. The second patient aged 25 years, para 2 was delivered by Caesarean section because she gradually developed focal neurological signs and became unconscious. Her death was due to cerebral infarction.

The other death was classified as fortuitous†. A 28 year old patient, para 4 died suddenly when she was ten weeks pregnant. Thrombosis of the right internal carotid artery with cerebral infarction was found at autopsy. There was no history of previous oral contraception.

* See page 7

Diabetes mellitus

Three deaths were attibuted to diabetes mellitus and were considered to be indirect.

One patient, a known diabetic, was admitted to hospital at about 11 weeks gestation in her first pregnancy with persistent nausea and vomiting. About 3 weeks later while still an in-patient she had a sudden cardiac arrest which was attributed to hypoglycaemia, because no other cause was found at autopsy.

The second patient also a primigravida was admitted to hospital as an emergency at the 25th week of pregnancy. She was vomiting and had diabetic ketosis and it was decided to terminate the pregnancy by hysterotomy. She died suddenly on the 13th post-operative day from bronchopneumonia. There had been some delay in identifying and treating the chest infection which had been the cause of the uncontrolled diabetes and this was considered to be an avoidable factor.

The third death occurred in a primigravida of 38 years with a longstanding history of diabetes and hypertension, who had been advised of the risks of pregnancy. She first attended the antenatal clinic at 17 weeks of pregnancy when her blood pressure was 170/120 mm Hg despite treatment with anti-hypertensive agents. She had refused a termination of pregnancy. At 37 weeks gestation arrangements were made for elective Caesarean section but she had a cardiac arrest during the induction of the anaesthetic and died. A post-mortem Caesarean section was performed and the baby was born alive but died after a few hours.

In addition a known diabetic died from pulmonary embolism 40 days after a normal delivery. This case was included in Chapter 4.

Encephalitis

There were two deaths from viral encephalitis, both of which were considered to be fortuitous†, one 10 weeks and the other 11 weeks after delivery.

Epilepsy

Three patients died from epilepsy.

One death was considered to be indirect. This patient who was para 3 aged 26 years, had had temporal lobe epilepsy since an attack of meningitis 16 years before. She died in status epilepticus following Caesarean section.

The other two deaths were fortuitous† and in known epileptics. One was found dead at home 22 days after delivery while the other drowned in her bath two months after delivery.

Diseases of gastrointestinal tract

(i) *Diaphragmatic hernia*

There were two indirect deaths in patients with diaphragmatic hernia.

One occurred in a woman para 7 aged 33 years, admitted to hospital at 26 weeks gestation with chest pain and vomiting. A diagnosis of diaphragmatic hernia was made. At 33 weeks she developed further chest pain, sudden respiratory embarrassment and circulatory collapse. At laparotomy gangrenous changes were found in the stomach. Gastroenterostomy and Caesarean section were carried out but the patient had a cardiac arrest during the operation and died. The other a woman with a known hiatus hernia was admitted to hospital complaining of abdominal pain and vomiting when 19 weeks pregnant. She improved with treatment but 5 days after admission she collapsed and died 5 hours later from rupture of the stomach.

(ii) *Spontaneous rupture of the stomach*

One patient, a primigravida, was found dead at home at 38 weeks gestation. The post-mortem report was inadequate but showed a rupture of an atrophic stomach near the oesophageal orifice. It was considered that this death might have been due to the gastro-oesophageal laceration— haemorrhage syndrome (Mallory-Weiss syndrome).

(iii) *Gastric ulceration*

A patient with an inevitable abortion at 22 weeks of pregnancy was examined under a general anaesthetic and the products of conception removed. She died suddenly 9 days later from haemorrhage from acute gastric ulceration. This was considered to be an indirect death.

(iv) *Gastroenteritis*

There was one fortuitous† death in the puerperium from viral gastro-enteritis.

(v) *Intestinal obstruction*

One patient was admitted at 26 weeks of pregnancy with acute intestinal obstruction. At laparotomy five days after admission she had a small bowel resection for gangrene due to adhesions resulting from a previous append-icectomy. The following day she had a spontaneous abortion. Ten days later she developed a faecal fistula and died suddenly a month later. The presence of the pregnancy was judged to have delayed the diagnosis. No autopsy was performed but this was considered to be an indirect death.

(vi) *Peritonitis*

One patient died from peritonitis secondary to intestinal obstruction caused by a foreign body. This followed a legal abortion and the case is counted in Chapter 5.

120

(vii) *Intussusception*

There was one death at 28 weeks of pregnancy in a patient who had an ileal intussusception associated with a papillary adenoma of the ileum. This was a fortuitous† death.

(viii) *Volvulus*

A death from volvulus occurred 8 months after a third elective lower segment Caesarean section. This death was classified as fortuitous†.

(ix) *Diseases of the colon*

Two patients died from Crohn's disease, and were considered to be indirect maternal deaths.

A woman aged 26 had been known to have Crohn's disease for six years. She was well during her pregnancy until she reached 24 weeks, when she had an acute recurrence which responded to treatment. She was admitted in preterm labour at 31 weeks gestation and was delivered of a live baby. On the 6th day of the puerperium she had a hemicolectomy and ileostomy for intestinal obstruction and generalized peritonitis. She died 3 days later. The second patient, aged 38, had Crohn's disease for 3 years. She had a normal pregnancy and delivery, being transferred home early from hospital. Four weeks after delivery she was referred back to hospital with loss of appetite, abdominal pain and a mass in the right iliac fossa. Despite surgical treatment she died 2 months after delivery from a paracolic abscess. This case is excluded under the international* definition of maternal death.

Two patients died from ulcerative colitis; one was an indirect and the other fortuitous†.

The first case, a primigravida aged 27 years had ulcerative colitis diagnosed about six months before she became pregnant. She was admitted at 27 weeks gestation with an exacerbation of her symptoms. She delivered spontaneously at 31 weeks but her condition then deteriorated and two days after delivery a colectomy with ileostomy was performed for bowel perforation and peritonitis. She died the following day. The second patient† died 14 weeks after a normal delivery when about to undergo colectomy for an exacerbation of ulcerative colitis which had not responded to medical treatment.

Hepatic failure

There were 2 cases of hepatic failure which were considered to be indirect.

One patient died eight months after delivery as the result of hepatic failure. She was well until 37 weeks gestation when nausea, vomiting and jaundice developed probably due to acute infective hepatitis. On admission the fetus was dead. The mother developed severe hepatic failure and cerebral necrosis and survived in an almost decerebrate state for eight months. This death would

* See page 7

be excluded under the international* definition of maternal deaths. The second patient aged 43 had a termination of pregnancy by hysterectomy at 15 weeks gestation. She developed jaundice 7 days later and died of acute hepatic necrosis 26 days after the operation.

Intracranial haemorrhage

There were 24 deaths from intracranial haemorrhage, excluding those from cerebral haemorrhage associated with the hypertensive diseases of pregnancy. None of these patients had had previous surgery for cerebral aneurysm but one had had a previous subarachnoid haemorrhage. All but one of these deaths were considered to be fortuitous†.

The one indirect obstetric death was that of a primigravida aged 24 years who was admitted at 30 weeks gestation with headache, paresis and loss of speech. A diagnosis of subarachnoid haemorrhage was made and at craniotomy an aneurysm of the pericallosal artery was clipped. Her condition remained fair for 48 hours and she then went into spontaneous labour complicated by placental abruption. She died 3 days after delivery, cerebral softening being found at autopsy.

Nine of the 23 fortuitous† deaths occurred during pregnancy, four due to subarachnoid and five to intracerebral haemorrhage. The haemorrhages occurred between 18 and 39 weeks of pregnancy. Two patients were delivered after the haemorrhage, one by Caesarean section and the other by forceps. Post-mortem examinations were performed in all cases, but only in two was positive evidence of an aneurysm found.

The remaining 14 women died from intracranial haemorrhage after delivery. Eight died after normal deliveries, and 6 of these deaths were within the first week and the others at 11 and 19 days after delivery. One woman who had an elective Caesarean section died 13 days after delivery. Post-mortem examinations revealed aneurysms in 5 of the 6 cases examined. In one of the cases where no autopsy was performed, ultra-sound scanning had revealed a massive intracranial haemorrhage. Five of the deaths occurred more than 6 weeks after delivery.

Kyphoscoliosis

A primigravida aged 33 years had severe kyphoscoliosis. She decided to take the risk of a pregnancy despite being warned of the risks. She went home 15 days after forceps delivery under local anaesthesia only to be readmitted 10 days later with increasing dyspnoea. A month later she developed respiratory failure and died 3 months after delivery. This was considered to be an indirect death.

* See page 7

122

Meningitis

One patient died of acute pneumococcal meningitis undelivered in the 38th week of her pregnancy. This was considered to be a fortuitous† death.

Neoplastic diseases

There were 33 deaths due to neoplastic disease. Thirty one were due to malignant disease, one to cerebral oedema caused by a benign tumour of the cerebral meninges and one to an extra-adrenal phaeochromocytoma. Eight of the deaths were considered to be indirect obstetric deaths and the other 25 fortuitous†. Of the fortuitous deaths, 11 were more than six weeks after delivery.

The sites of the tumours were as follows:—

Site of tumour	ICD number	Number of patients	Age at death (years)
Indirect			
ICD Code 648 with additional Code:—			
Breast ⎰ carcinoma	174	2	33,36
⎱ lymphosarcoma	200.1	2	31
Ovary sarcoma	183.0	1	15
Melanoma	172	3	25,27,32
Phaeochromocytoma	227.8	1	24
Fortuitous			
Oesophagus	150	2	31,42
Stomach	151	3	28,32,33
Colon	153	3	24,25,33
Liver	155	2	25,29
Bronchus	162	1	36
Melanoma	172	2	22,29
Cerebrum	191	9	14,17,24, 26,27,27, 27,34,42
Disseminated malignant neoplasm	199	2	33,44
Cerebral meninges	225.2	1	29

There was one indirect death attributed to phaeochromocytoma. The patient who had had a previous Caesarean section for disproportion 3 years previously was well until 38 weeks gestation. She then developed hypertension, the blood pressure rising to between 160/110 and 190/120 mm Hg over several days without proteinuria. At Caesarean section there was respiratory difficulty and after delivery a diagnosis of pulmonary oedema was made, the blood

123

pressure fell and she died later the same day. At post-mortem examination an extra-adrenal phaeochromocytoma was found attached to the abdominal aorta.

There was one death from choriocarcinoma which occurred within one year of the causal pregnancy and is discussed in Chapter 13.

Pituitary infarction

A primigravida aged 30 years with a twin pregnancy was admitted for 10 days rest at 35 weeks gestation complaining of tiredness and vomiting. She was readmitted in early labour at 37 weeks with a history of nausea and polyuria and the fetal hearts could not be heard. She appeared toxic and dehydrated and her serum electrolytes were grossly abnormal. One and a half hours after vaginal delivery she became unconscious and was transferred to the intensive care unit. After further investigation a diagnosis of diabetes insipidus was made and despite treatment she died 4 days after delivery. At autopsy there was a recent infarction of the anterior and posterior lobes of the pituitary of undetermined cause. This was considered to be an indirect death.

Respiratory diseases

(i) *Asthma*

There were 4 deaths ascribed to asthma and one anaesthetic death, described in Chapter 8, where the patient's asthmatic condition was considered to have contributed to her death.

Three of the deaths were classified as indirect. In 2 of these anaesthesia was considered to have been a contributory factor, both cases had epidural analgesia in labour and emergency Caesarean section. Each patient developed severe bronchospasm during the operation and are discussed in Chapter 8. The third patient, aged 30 years para 2, had developed asthma after her first pregnancy. She had had asthmatic attacks during her final pregnancy but refused to take any regular medication on a preventive basis. At 38 weeks gestation she was admitted to hospital in status asthmaticus which responded to treatment and she had a normal labour and delivery. She was well when she went home but 17 days after delivery she had a severe asthmatic attack and died before her general practitioner could attend her. The patient's lack of co-operation with treatment has been regarded as an avoidable factor.

There was one other fortuitous† death which was in an asthmatic patient eight months after delivery.

(ii) *Bronchiectasis*

One patient, para 2 aged 25 years had had bronchiectasis since childhood. When she was 16 weeks pregnant she had 3 episodes of haemoptysis in one day and was admitted to hospital where she died after a massive

124

haemorrhage within 24 hours. The chest physician was of the opinion that she had deliberately failed to obtain treatment earlier for her chest infection due to her reluctance to take any medication during pregnancy. This death was regarded as indirect.

(iii) Pneumonia

In 12 cases of maternal death the cause was pneumonia. In 5 of these patients the infection was present at the time of abortion or delivery and a causal factor of premature labour. These have been classified as indirect deaths.

The cases and causative organisms were as follows:—

Disease	Causative organisms	ICD number	Number of patients	Age at death (years)
Indirect				
ICD Code 647.8 with additional code				
Bronchopneumonia and myocarditis	Parainfluenza virus	480.2	1	31
Bronchopneumonia	Staphylococcus	482.4	1	30
Pneumonia and lung abscesses	Staphylococcus	487.4	1	26
Lobar pneumonia and empyema	*Escherichia Coli*	482.8	1	17
Bronchopneumonia	Influenzal	487.0	1	27
Fortuitous†				
Pneumonia	Varicella	052	2	24,25
Bronchopneumonia	Viral	480.8	1	24
Bronchopneumonia	Staphylococcus	482.4	1	22
Post-influenzal pneumonia	Staphylococcus	487.0	2	23,28
Lobar pneumonia and septicaemia	*Escherichia Coli*	482.8	1	34

(iv) Interstitial pulmonary emphysema

One indirect death involved a patient who had a Caesarean section at 37 weeks of pregnancy. She apparently recovered well until the 9th post-operative day when she was thought to have had a pulmonary embolism and despite treatment she had a cardiac arrest. At post-mortem examination there was no evidence of embolism and she was found to have died from pulmonary interstitial emphysema.

Renal diseases

(i) *Pyelonephritis*

There were 2 cases of pyelonephritis, one indirect and one fortuitous†.

The indirect death occurred in a patient who concealed her pregnancy until she was at term. She died of gram-negative septicaemia secondary to acute suppurative pyelonephritis. There was one other case of pyelonephritis associated with a renal calculus which was considered to be fortuitous†.

(ii) *Renal failure*

There were two indirect deaths due to renal failure.

The first patient died from chronic recurrent urinary tract infection. The other patient aged 29 years, died 48 days after a spontaneous abortion at 26 weeks of pregnancy. She died from renal cortical infarction and hypertension, but the abortion was not thought to have been a causal factor. This case would be excluded under the international* definition of maternal death.

Septicaemia

There were 2 deaths from septicaemia, one indirect and one fortuitous†.

The indirect death occurred in a patient who developed varicella and threatened to abort at the 10th week of pregnancy. Because of this she was admitted to hospital and her condition deteriorated very rapidly and she died within 12 hours. Death was due to viraemia and septicaemia, β *Haemolytic streptococcus* (Group A) as well as viruses being isolated from many sites in the body. As the source of the streptococcal infection was not known this had been considered an indirect death.

The other patient died from septicaemia due to β *Haemolytic streptococcus* (Group A) and *Streptococcus pneumoniae.* Although her death occurred 14 days after her delivery the source of the infection was thought to be from an infected graze on her elbow, and not from a uterine infection. This was considered to be a fortuitous† death.

Sudden death of unknown cause after the puerperium

Four deaths occurred more than 42 days after delivery and have been classified as fortuitous† as no satisfactory cause of death was found.

One patient, para 2 aged 30 years, died 43 days after a normal pregnancy, delivery and puerperium. She was found dead at home. Post-mortem examination, including histological examination, failed to reveal any convincing cause of death.

An apparently similar death occurred in a primigravida aged 20 who collapsed and died at home 46 days after a normal pregnancy, delivery and puerperium. Post-mortem examination revealed no conclusive cause of death, but no information was available on histological or toxicological examinations.

* See page 7

A West Indian woman aged 21 years collapsed and died in the street 3 months after a normal second pregnancy and delivery. She had a sickle cell trait with haemoglobin A and S which was not considered to have been significant. Despite a detailed post-mortem examination and histological study no cause of death was found.

Another woman aged 22 years had a normal second pregnancy, delivery and puerperium. Four months later she developed diarrhoea and vomiting. Her general practitioner thought she had a viral infection and she deteriorated suddenly after 3 days of illness and was sent to hospital. She had a cardiac arrest in the ambulance and could not be resuscitated. Post-mortem examination suggested myocarditis, but unfortunately no histological, bacteriological or toxicological examination was made.

Sudden unnatural deaths

These deaths are grouped together and include cases of suicide, cases where the coroners' courts returned open or misadventure verdicts or verdicts of accidental death, and two cases of manslaughter. Road traffic accidents have been considered separately.

Suicide

There were 18 cases of suicide, one antenatal and 17 postnatal. Seven of these were considered to be fortuitous† as they appeared to have been unrelated to pregnancy or childbirth. Six of these occurred between 2 and 11 months after delivery, 5 of the women having had long psychiatric histories. Two of the women were Asian.

Eleven of the deaths from suicide have been classified as indirect although 5 would be excluded under the international* definition of maternal death as they occurred more than 6 weeks after delivery. However in each of these 5 cases there had been evidence of depression during pregnancy or the puerperium and all had been under treatment before their deaths. One had been refused termination of an unwanted pregnancy and adoption was being arranged.

In 2 of the remaining cases the women had appeared to their families and medical attendants to be only mildly anxious about feeding difficulties and their suicides were quite unexpected. Another had asked for her baby to be taken into temporary foster care but killed herself despite this having been arranged.

One single girl managed to conceal both her pregnancy and a stillbirth at home and then took an overdose of salicylates and drowned herself. Another single girl was discharged after delivery to stay with friends and took an overdose on the 10th day. She returned home and killed herself 4 days later with an overdose of amitriptyline.

* See page 7

127

An Asian woman had refused contraceptive advice after her first pregnancy but became depressed and killed herself and her baby five months later, when she was again 14 weeks pregnant.

Open verdict or misadventure verdict

There were 14 cases in which the coroner gave an open or a misadventure verdict.

Ten of these cases were considered to be fortuitous† and the deaths were either related to family or social problems or in 2 cases occurred in known drug addicts.

In 4 cases it was considered that the death was an indirect death. One single girl concealed her pregnancy and took an overdose of salicylates at 23 weeks gestation. However it was decided that this had been done to get rid of the pregnancy and was not primarily a suicide attempt.

Another woman, with a twin pregnancy, took an overdose of salicylates at 36 weeks. This caused an antepartum haemorrhage and disseminated intravascular coagulation. The twins were delivered by forceps and both were stillborn, the mother dying from respiratory failure 19 days postpartum.

The other two cases would both be excluded under the international* definition of maternal death. They were both under treatment for puerperal depression and died between 3 and 5 months after delivery.

Accidental deaths

There were six accidental deaths (excluding road traffic accidents). Three were classified as fortuitous†, one of which was by drowning, one by accidental carbon monoxide poisoning and one was a death in a railway accident.

There were 3 indirect deaths. In one of these very serious burns in a domestic fire caused a spontaneous abortion at 26 weeks of pregnancy. Another woman died from the inhalation of smoke in a domestic fire. A post-mortem Caesarean section was performed but the baby was stillborn. The third death would be excluded under the international* definition of maternal death, it involved a patient who was seen and treated for depression by her general practitioner 6 weeks after delivery. Two days later she was found wandering at night and died of exposure. The drugs identified at post-mortem examination had been prescribed and had been taken only in therapeutic dosage.

Road traffic accidents

There were 6 deaths from road traffic accidents and all have been classified as fortuitous†. In 5 cases death due to multiple injuries occurred at the time of the accident. Three of these women were pregnant, two at 14 to 16 weeks of

* See page 7

128

pregnancy, and one at 38 weeks. Two women died 8 and 10 months, respectively, after delivery. The sixth woman was also pregnant at about 36 weeks gestation. She was involved in a collision in a car while wearing a seat belt. On admission she was not at first thought to be seriously injured, but she had a traumatic placental abruption, the uterus being hard and the fetal heart inaudible. She went into spontaneous labour and there was evidence of disseminated intravascular coagulation. Despite appropriate treatment she became comatose 6 hours after delivery with evidence of increased intracerebral pressure. She was transferred to a neurosurgical unit, and at operation was found to have a massive intracerebral haemorrhage, and died 11 days after the accident.

Manslaughter

There were two cases of manslaughter. One died by strangulation at 22 weeks gestation, and the other by stabbing at 19 weeks gestation. These were classified as fortuitous† deaths.

15. Post-mortem examinations

In the last report which covered the years 1973 – 1975, the Chief Medical Officer wrote in his preface

'The importance of accurate diagnosis of the cause of death becomes greater as the number of deaths diminish. Port-mortem examinations were carried out in 344 out of the 390 deaths investigated, but the authors and the regional assessors have all expressed concern that the reports available were not all as helpful as they might have been. The assessors need full details of the post-mortem and all histological examinations. More discussion between the clinicians and the pathologists as to the cause of death at the time of the examination might help to elucidate some of the problems.'

In some cases lack of detail in the post-mortem report and in other cases apparently inadequate post-mortem examination made it difficult to assess the cause of death with accuracy. For example, in 6 out of 36 autopsies the source of the pulmonary embolus was not looked for and microscopic examination of the lungs was omitted in several cases of suspected amniotic fluid embolism. Post-mortem examination can contribute so much to the ultimate solution of the reasons behind a maternal death, that it should be completely performed and recorded. Pathologists have a responsibility to support their clinical colleagues by undertaking searching autopsies, which must involve the carrying out of all the appropriate investigations, macroscopic, microscopic and laboratory if required to establish the cause of death.

In preparing this report the Department's Consultant Adviser in Histopathology was invited at the beginning of 1980 to join with the Advisers in Obstetrics and Gynaecology and in Anaesthesia, to discuss with them those reports in which essential autopsy information appeared to be lacking or inadequate and how the standard might be improved. No detailed retrospective histopathological study has been attempted as the autopsies concerned had already been completed and little more detailed information could be obtained, but certain general observations are pertinent.

Autopsies associated with childbearing fall into two categories. The majority are for medico-legal purposes and are done on the instruction of the Coroner who nominates a medical practitioner to perform them. This may be a histopathologist with special forensic skill or one with special experience in maternal deaths but more commonly it is a consultant histopathologist who has no specialized experience in the maternal field. Rarely, it may be a junior pathologist in training or a medical practitioner not primarily trained as a histopathologist and without the necessary supportive technical and laboratory facilities. A minority of deaths are not referred to the Coroner. In these autopsy may be omitted or be performed either by a consultant pathologist, with or without specialized experience in maternal deaths, or, more commonly, by junior staff in training and with different degrees of supervision.

In the present report, out of 227 true obstetric deaths 194 were referred to the Coroner and had autopsies performed; of the remaining 33, 12 had no autopsy and in a further 3 no autopsy report could be obtained. In the 200 associated deaths 133 were referred to the Coroner and 44 had no autopsy performed; in a further 2 no autopsy report was available.

The pathologist who performs a maternal autopsy whether or not it is for the coroner has two distinct responsibilities. First, particularly in coroner's cases, he must try to determine accurately the cause of death; second he must try to determine the chain of events which led up to death and to link these with the clinical history so that an explanation as well as a cause can be given. All the abnormalities discovered have to be carefully recorded. The requirements for a good autopsy include an adequate clinical history available in advance, not only with the incidents recorded which led to the death but also the temporal relationships of these.

The circumstances surrounding the arrangements for coroners' autopsies are often less than ideal. They are often undertaken in a mortuary at a distance from the maternity unit so that clinico-pathological communication is poor; they are performed to discover causes of death rather than to make clinico-pathological assessments and histological examinations are often not attempted. Inadequate histories may mean that careful search is not made for particular features or causes features to be missed or mis-interpreted; for example unless it is known that inhalation of gastric contents has occurred previously, inflammation of trachea and bronchi may be wrongly attributed to trauma during endotracheal intubation. The autopsy examination should always include a search for macroscopic features peculiarly associated with maternal death such as venous sinus thrombosis in the skull or evidence of air or amniotic fluid embolus. It must always be supported by adequate histo-logical examination and other laboratory procedures where appropriate and it is particularly important that all apparently normal organs should be clearly described as 'normal on examination' or 'unexamined'. If a stillborn child and/or a placenta are available these should be examined by the pathologist who performs the maternal autopsy or a report on them should be made available to him. In some autopsies no clear cause of death can at once be determined; in some of these subsequent investigations will confirm a pro-visional diagnosis, e.g. histopathological studies can confirm suspected amniotic fluid embolism. The pathologist must on occasion be prepared to say that he cannot determine a cause of death, and he must always sample and retain those tissues and other material which might confirm the macroscopic diagnosis he has made. Finally he owes a duty to his obstetric and anaesthetic colleagues and most of all to the husband of the patient to provide as far as he can an adequate explanation for the death which has occurred.

Some general suggestions can be given as to how the value of post-mortem examination can be improved.

1. As adequate history must be available in advance and the clinicians con-cerned should attend the autopsy whenever possible.

2. Autopsies on these patients should be regarded as specialized investi-gations. Coroners should be encouraged to consider maternal deaths as

falling within a special category and as far as possible to ask pathologists with special interest or expertise in the field to perform them. They should never be performed by practitioners without training in histopathology and advice should be available for those pathologists without special experience.
3. Pathologists, particularly those specializing in medico-legal autopsies should be encouraged to preserve appropriate blocks of tissue, other than those required solely to establish a cause of death even if they do not examine these themselves. Such material is essential for subsequent study.

The recent appointment of Regional Advisors in Pathology able to give special advice in the light of their own experience should have considerable value in raising local standards where these are below what is desirable.

An article giving guidelines on the performance of autopsies on patients whose death is associated with childbirth is to be published in the Journal of Clinical Pathology in the autumn of 1982.

16. Booking arrangements for women in the enquiry series

The arrangements made for confinement by the 427 women included in the 1976–78 enquiry have been studied. Initially 280 (65.6%) of the women were booked for delivery in consultant obstetric units a decrease of 2.1% compared with the 1973–75 series. Fifty two (12.2%) were booked for general practitioner units and 6 (1.4%) were booked for domiciliary confinements. Of the 427 maternal deaths 84 (19.7%) of the women had made no booking at the time of death and for a further 2 (0.5%) no booking was known of at the time of the enquiry. However 36 (42.9%) of these 84 women died before the 13th week of pregnancy before booking arrangements could be confirmed and a few others had requested termination of their pregnancies.

Table 16.1 shows an analysis of the initial booking arrangements for the last 3 triennia.

Table 16.1: *Initial booking arrangements in 1970–72, 1973–75 and 1976–78 enquiries*

Initial booking arrangements	1970–72		1973–75		1976–78	
	No	%	No	%	No	%
Domiciliary	44	7.3	10	2.6	6	1.4
General practioner unit (i) separate (ii) with consultant unit	67	11.1	38	9.7	13⎫ 39⎭ 52	3.0⎫ 12.1 9.1⎭
Private nursing home	3	0.5	1	0.3	1	0.2
Consultant unit	319	52.6	264	67.7	280	65.6
Services Hospital	4	0.7	2	0.5	2	0.5
No booking made	153	25.2	71	18.2	84	19.7
No information about booking	16	2.6	4	1.0	2	0.5

133

Table 16.2 gives details of the place of delivery of births in triennia from 1967–1978. There has been a continuously rising trend in the proportion of births in hospital and a decrease in domiciliary confinement.

Table 16.2: *Hospital and domiciliary maternity services*

		1967–69	1970–72	1973–75	1976–78
Total births	Number	2,484,004	2,322,124	1,940,689	1,766,169
Live births	Number	2,448,974	2,293,081	1,919,283	1,749,947
Still births	Number	35,030	29,043	21,406	16,222
Births					
In NHS hospital	Number	1,951,231	2,023,413	1,818,017	1,706,677
In other hospitals[1]	Number	52,380	42,209	32,407	22,599
At home[2]	Number	480,393	256,502	90,265	35,215
Total births					
In NHS hospitals	per cent	78.6	87.1	93.7	96.6
In all hospitals	per cent	80.7	89.0	95.3	97.9
NHS hospital					
Consultant obst. beds	Number	—	55,072	54,462	51,507
GP obstetric beds	Number	—	15,297	14,179	11,613
Domiciliary midwives					
Deliveries attended	Number	471,132	278,344	160,042	107,288
Early transfer cases[3]	Number	1,029,849	1,340,775	1,419,235	1,501,251

[1] Births in non NHS hospitals and maternity homes.

[2] Includes births occurring in homes for unmarried mothers, remand homes, reception centres etc.

[3] Patients transferred from hospital before the tenth day and attended by domiciliary midwives.

Domiciliary midwives do most of their work outside hospital in the community but are often based in a hospital, and may attend deliveries not only at home but also in general practitioner units and some consultant units. This accounts for an increasing discrepancy in recent years between the number of deliveries they attend and the numbers of births at home.

Table 16.3 gives the estimated proportion of maternities taking place at home in the 3 triennia 1970–72, 1973–75 and 1976–78 for each hospital region. The proportion of domicilary deliveries was reduced in all the regions in successive years.

Table 16.3: *Proportion of maternities (estimated) confined at home in 1970–1978*

Regional Health Authority*	1970–72	1973–75	1976–78
Northern	7.8	3.2	1.4
Yorkshire	11.1	4.5	2.3
Trent	14.0	6.1	2.3
East Anglian	17.8	8.2	3.5
N.W. Thames	9.8	4.4	2.0
N.E. Thames	14.2	6.4	2.8
S.E. Thames	12.9	6.0	2.8
S.W. Thames	6.0	2.6	1.2
Wessex	10.3	3.1	1.5
Oxford	6.8	2.1	1.0
South Western	7.2	2.7	1.5
West Midlands	12.8	4.8	2.2
Mersey	9.8	4.2	1.9
North Western	11.2	5.0	2.0
Wales	5.2	2.1	1.5
England and Wales	10.7	4.5	2.0

* Note the reorganization of the National Health Service occurred in 1974. After reorganization the 14 Regions of England were renamed, but there were not very large alterations in the boundaries so that the deaths in the Regions can be compared in the different triennia without significant distortion.

Women with no booking arrangements

The duration of pregnancy at the time of death or delivery of the 84 women with no booking arrangements is shown in Table 16.4.

Table 16.4: *Duration of pregnancy at death or delivery of the women with no booking arrangements*

Duration of pregnancy in weeks	True deaths	Associated deaths	Total deaths
6 or less	7	1	8
7–12	17	3	20
13–20	17	10	27
21–28	1	6	7
29–36	4	1	5
37+	3	3	6
Not stated	9	2	11
Total	58	26	84

Of the 84 women for whom no booking arrangements were made it is estimated that 8 died on or before the 6th week of pregnancy, 20 died between

135

the 7th and 12th week, 34 between the 13th and 28th week, 11 after the 28th week, and in 11 the duration of pregnancy was not stated

An analysis of these 5 groups shows the following causes of death:—

1. Duration of pregnancy: 6 weeks or less
   Cause of death:-

Ectopic pregnancy	7
Other causes	1
	8

2. Duration of pregnancy: 7–12 weeks
   Cause of death:-

Abortion — legal	2
other	1
Ectopic pregnancy	4
Pulmonary embolism	5
Associated with anaesthesia	4
Other causes	4
	20

Although there were considered to be avoidable factors associated with some of these deaths, the fact that no booking had been made was in no case considered to have been a contributory cause. Three died from associated causes.

3. Duration of pregnancy: 13–28 weeks
   Cause of death:-

Abortion — legal	6
other	4
Ectopic pregnancy	1
Pulmonary embolism	3
Associated with anaesthesia	1
Other causes	19
	34

Of the 23 women dying from causes other than abortion or ectopic pregnancy, 16 died undelivered. Eleven of these died from associated causes. In two of these cases avoidable factors were attributed to the patients neither of whom had sought medical care during their pregnancy. A single girl concealed her pregnancy and then took an overdose of salicylates, apparently with the hope of getting rid of the pregnancy at 23 weeks gestation. Another patient aged 41 years with long standing rheumatic heart disease did not get in touch with her general practitioner until she had to be admitted as an emergency at sixteen weeks of pregnancy and died 3 days later.

Three women died from pulmonary embolism at 14, 15 and 20 weeks. The first had attended her general practitioner and a pregnancy test had been performed but no booking arrangements made. She was admitted to hospital as an emergency with abdominal pain. The second patient, a para 4 aged 41 years died suddenly at home at 15 weeks of pregnancy having had no antenatal care. Unfortunately no information was obtainable from her general practitioner about her previous pregnancies or medical history. The third patient was a single non-resident woman working in this country, who had attended her general practitioner and a hospital for varicose veins before she became pregnant, but had apparently made no attempt to obtain antenatal care. She died suddenly at home at 20 weeks of pregnancy.

One patient died from cerebral haemorrhage due to severe pre-eclampsia at 24 weeks gestation in her first pregnancy. She had attended a midwife twice at 14 and 16 weeks of pregnancy but had then moved house and had not apparently attended a new general practitioner to arrange for antenatal care or for booking. She was admitted as an emergency with two weeks history of headache and vomiting and died the same day.

4. Duration of pregnancy: more than 28 weeks.
    Cause of death:-

Hypertensive diseases of pregnancy	3
Puerperal sepsis	2
Haemorrhage	1
Cardiac disease	1
Associated with anaesthesia	1
Other causes	3
	11

Brief details of the 11 women who had made no arrangements for delivery, although at or past the 28th week of pregnancy are as follows:

(i) Primigravida aged 18 years a concealed illegitimate pregnancy. She had been attending her general practitioner for increasing weight and oedema of her ankles, but the pregnancy was not detected. She was found dead at home one morning from asphyxia having apparently had an eclamptic fit. She may have been in early labour as her membranes had ruptured.

(ii) Primigravida aged 20 years, a concealed illegitimate pregnancy. She committed suicide by drowning, having given birth at term to a stillborn infant unattended at home.

(iii) Primigravida aged 21 years, a concealed illegitimate pregnancy. She was found unconscious at home at about 36 weeks of pregnancy. Her blood pressure was 250/140 mm Hg on admission and she was treated for eclampsia. Labour was induced and she was delivered of a stillborn fetus. She was treated for renal failure but died 5 days after delivery from cerebral haemorrhage and pneumonia.

(iv) Primigravida aged 29 years, a married woman with a long psychiatric history who had no antenatal care. She was admitted at term and had a normal delivery. She discharged herself from hospital on the day of delivery and disappeared to be found dead out of doors two weeks later as a result of exposure and aspirin overdosage.

(v)   Para 2 aged 19 years had attended her general practitioner on one occasion during her pregnancy but did not keep her hospital booking appointment despite 2 reminders. She concealed her pregnancy from her family until after her marriage and while away on holiday in a caravan was delivered of a stillborn abnormal baby of about 38 weeks gestation, with no professional help. She was finally admitted to hospital 2 days later and died of septicaemia.

(vi)   Para 2 aged 25 years had no antenatal care. She was admitted in labour and required a Caesarean section but she died as a result of anaesthetic difficulties from Mendelson's syndrome.

(vii)   Para 3 aged 25 years had no antenatal care and by deliberate choice had a delivery at home assisted only by her husband. The baby was a full term normal stillbirth. The mother died 3 days after delivery from puerperal sepsis.

(viii)   Para 5 aged 26 years had no antenatal care. She was admitted as an emergency, not having seen her doctor, complaining of headache and vomiting at about 34 weeks of pregnancy. Her blood pressure was 200/110 mm Hg and she was treated for severe pre-eclampsia and labour was induced. She had an eclamptic fit before delivery of a stillborn infant. She died from cerebral haemorrhage 2 days later.

(ix)   Para 5 aged 33 years concealed her pregnancy because she knew she had a lump in her breast and was afraid of being advised to have the pregnancy terminated. She eventually went to see her doctor at about 36 weeks of pregnancy and was admitted to hospital and was delivered by forceps. She died 13 days later from metastases from carcinoma of the breast.

(x)   Para 7 aged 36 years of Asian origin had no antenatal care and she was admitted as an emergency in the second stage of labour. She discharged herself 24 hours after delivery and died at home 3 weeks after delivery from pulmonary oedema consequent on mitral stenosis.

(xi)   Para 11 aged 40 years also of Asian origin had no antenatal care until she was admitted with antepartum haemorrhage at 27 weeks of pregnancy. Two weeks after admission she developed placental abruption and was delivered by Caesarean section, but died from the effects of haemorrhage.

In the 5 cases of concealed pregnancy the failure of the woman to seek antenatal care is regarded as an avoidable factor.

5.   Duration of pregnancy not stated
      Cause of death:-

Ectopic pregnancy	7
Associated with anaesthesia	1
Haemorrhage	1
Puerperal sepsis	1
Other	1
	11

Three of these patients died apparently after the 28th week of pregnancy, and details of these cases are as follows:-

(i)   Primigravida aged 17 years a concealed illegitimate pregnancy. She was admitted to a medical ward at about the 36th week of pregnancy with lobar pneumonia. She went into labour and was delivered of a stillborn baby the day after admission, and died later the same day.

(ii)   Primigravida aged 41 years a married woman who was very obese and concealed her pregnancy from her husband. She complained of backache and a cough and was seen at home by a general practitioner. She died at home the following day from septicaemia and acute suppurative pyelonephritis. At post-mortem examination a macerated stillbirth was found in the vagina. She was thought to have been almost at term.

(iii)   A para 7 aged 33 years had no antenatal care. She and her husband decided to deliver the baby at home. An ambulance was called about 14 hours after delivery when the baby had died, but the mother refused hospital admission. About 4 hours later a police surgeon was called and sent her into hospital where on arrival she was dead from postpartum haemorrhage.

Women booked for domiciliary confinement

There were 6 deaths among women initially booked for home confinement during 1976−78, compared with 10 in 1973−75 and 44 in 1970−72.

Of the 6 cases, only 3 were actually delivered at home. The first case was a para 2 aged 31 years who had a normal delivery at 38 weeks with an episiotomy. Forty eight hours after delivery she was admitted to hospital with lower abdominal pain, bleeding and infection of the episiotomy wound. She died 7 hours after admission from haemolytic streptococcal septicaemia.

The second case was also a para 2 aged 29 years. She had a normal full term delivery at home. She developed deep vein thrombosis with episodes of breathlessness but was not admitted to hospital until almost 4 weeks after delivery when she was seriously ill. She died later the same day despite pulmonary embolectomy.

The third patient a para aged 29 years died at home undelivered in labour at 43 weeks of pregnancy. She had fits during the second stage of labour and the midwife called the Emergency Obstetric Service. The mother and baby were already dead when it reached the home. The cause of death was given as air embolism but unfortunately no histological examination was made.

The fourth patient aged 31 years para 3 died in hospital from influenzal viral pneumonia which she developed on the day of delivery. She was treated at home by her general practitioner with antibiotics, but was admitted to hospital eight days after delivery when her condition deteriorated and the following day she died despite treatment.

The other two patients booked for home confinement, both had their bookings transferred to a consultant unit before delivery.

Women booked for delivery in general practitioner maternity units

For the purposes of this report a general practitioner unit is defined as a place equipped for normal obstetrics but where there is no resident doctor. These do not in fact form a homogenous group since they are sited differently some being within or adjacent to hospital consultant obstetric units some separated from them by a considerable distance. An attempt has been made in this report to distinguish these general practitioner units which were apparently quite separate geographically from any consultant obstetric unit or any acute hospital services and the others where some closer connection was apparent. This has had to be rather an arbitrary division as the degree of co-ordination and support between general practitioner units and their local consultant units is as important to the obstetric service as the physical distance between them.

There were 52 deaths among women initially booked for confinement in a general practitioner unit of whom 13 were booked for 'separate' units as described above.

Table 16.5 shows the deaths of women by age and parity who were booked for delivery in general practitioner units in 1976–78. If it is considered that it is suitable for general practitioner units to book for delivery primigravidae under 30 years and women in their 2nd, 3rd or 4th pregnancy under 35 years then it will be seen from Table 16.5 that only 3 women out of the 52 would be considered to have been wrongly booked for delivery at a general practitioner unit on the grounds of age and parity alone. None of these were booked at a separate general practitioner unit.

Table 16.5: *The number of deaths of women by age and parity booked for delivery in general practitioner maternity units, 1976 – 78*

	Age (years)	Parity					
		1	2	3	4	5–9	Total
'Separate' Units	16–19	—	—	—	—	—	—
	20–24	5	—	—	—	—	5
	25–29	4	1	1	—	—	6
	30–34	—	2	—	—	—	2
	35–39	—	—	—	—	—	—
	Total	9	3	1	0	0	13
'Other' GP units	16–19	4	—	—	—	—	4
	20–24	8	1	—	—	—	9
	25–29	3	8	1	1	—	13
	30–34	1	4	3	2	1	11
	35–39	—	—	1	—	1	2
	Total	16	13	5	3	2	39
	Total	25	16	6	3	2	52

Fifteen of the 52 women had their bookings transferred to a consultant unit during the course of their pregnancy (Table 16.6) Eight of the transferred bookings took place at or after the 36th week of pregnancy. In one case the failure to book initially for a consultant unit was considered to have been an avoidable factor in a patient with a history of ulcerative colitis. Another case of twin pregnancy had her booking transferred to a consultant unit and when an emergency occurred in labour the obstetric registrar and blood supplies had to come from a larger unit 10 miles away.

The sequence of events in the cases of the 52 women who died is summarized in Table 16.6.

Table 16.6: *Deaths of women booked for delivery in general practitioner maternity units—sequence of events*

Booking, delivery, death	Number of cases	Unavoidable deaths	Deaths with avoidable factors
Initial booking for general practitioner unit	52	35	17
a. 'Separate' unit	13	3	10
b. 'Other' unit	39	32	7
Booking transferred to a consultant unit during pregnancy	15	10	5
Admitted to hospital unbooked before delivery:			
1. To obstetric consultant unit			
Died undelivered	1	1	—
delivered	12	3	9
Died more than 6 weeks after delivery from an associated cause	3	3	—
2. To non-obstetric consultant unit			
Died undelivered	4	3	1
delivered	2	2	—
Died at home, undelivered	3	3	—
Died in GP unit	—	—	—
Delivered in GP unit:			
1. Died after transfer to consultant unit	2	1	1
2. Died at home in puerperium	1	1	—
3. Died more than 6 weeks after delivery			
a. from obstetric cause	2	2	—
b. from associated cause	7	6	1

It is important to note that out of the 52 cases initially booked for GP units 25 were primigravidae of whom 9 were booked at the 'separate' GP units and 16 at the 'other' units.

Women booked at separate GP units

Five of the 9 primigravidae booked at the separate GP units developed eclampsia and in four of these cases the general practitioners responsible for their antenatal care were considered to have been at fault in not referring them for consultant advice when early signs of pre-eclampsia developed. They were all finally transferred to consultant units for delivery. In the fifth case the booking and antenatal care was transferred to the consultant at 37 weeks gestation but the patient was not admitted until she was 2 weeks overdue when her blood pressure was 140/90 mm Hg and she developed eclampsia before labour could be induced. All these patients with eclampsia died from cerebral haemorrhage.

Another primigravida booked at a separate maternity unit developed epileptic fits when 16 weeks pregnant. She was treated by her general practitioner but not referred for a consultant opinion. She had a normal delivery, but was readmitted to hospital 3 weeks later, when a cerebral tumour was found at craniotomy. It was considered that earlier referral and investigation might have affected the outcome.

Another patient with a history of ulcerative colitis should not have been booked for delivery in a separate maternity unit, although her booking was transferred at 29 weeks gestation when her colitis had deteriorated. She died following a premature delivery at 31 weeks.

The deaths of the two other primigravidae and the four multiparae were unrelated to their booking arrangements at separate units.

Women booked at other GP units

Of the 16 primigravidae originally booked at other GP units 11 of their deaths were due to associated causes and in only one case was the booking considered to have been an avoidable factor in the death. This patient, who was only 152 cm in height was referred for a consultant opinion when the fetal head was not engaged at 38 weeks of pregnancy. The booking was not changed and she had to be transferred to the consultant unit in labour with delay in the second stage. She had a forceps delivery and later required anaesthesia for evacuation of a haematoma. She died following an anaesthetic complication. Another primigravida aged 32 years had her booking transferred to a consultant unit before delivery.

Of the 23 multiparae originally booked at other general practitioner units, 15 died from associated causes. Three of the true obstetric deaths were wrongly booked on grounds of age and parity alone. A para 5 aged 32 years, and six years after her last delivery, developed hypertension of 130/98 mm Hg and proteinuria at 38 weeks of pregnancy but was not referred for consultant advice. At term she had an antepartum haemorrhage and intrauterine death occurred which led to the development of a coagulation defect and she died following a massive postpartum haemorrhage.

A para 7 aged 38 years was booked for a general practitioner unit though her doctor noted that he had intended to transfer her booking to the consultant unit before delivery. She developed pre-eclampsia, was admitted to the consultant unit and died from coronary thrombosis two weeks after a Caesarean section.

The third patient, para 3 aged 35 years, had her booking transferred to a consultant unit at term.

Another patient, para 2, aged 25 years, should not have been booked for a general practitioner unit because at the time of her first delivery, pelvimetry had revealed a degree of contracted pelvis. She had also had a moderate postpartum haemorrhage.

Although the criteria for booking a patient in a general practitioner unit are well defined there is still a failure to appreciate that the decision needs to be reviewed regularly throughout the pregnancy, particularly in relation to hypertensive diseases of pregnancy.

Tables 16.7 and 16.8 show the number of deaths of women by age and parity booked for delivery in general practitioner units from 1970–78 and the proportion which had avoidable factors. In the absence of reliable information about all the total number of women who were booked for delivery in these units during these years it is not possible to calculate a death rate.

Table 16.7: *Deaths of women by age, booked for delivery in general practitioner maternity units 1970–1978 and the proportion with avoidable factors*

Age (years)	All deaths	Deaths with avoidable factor present	
		Number	Proportion of all deaths (per cent)
< 19	14	6	42.9
20–24	46	14	30.4
25–29	58	23	39.7
30–34	30	13	43.3
35–39	9	2	22.2
40–44	—	—	—
45+	—	—	—
All	157	58	36.9

Table 16.8: *Deaths of women, by parity*, booked for delivery in general practitioner maternity units, 1970–78 and the proportion with avoidable factors*

Parity	All deaths	Deaths with avoidable factor present	
		Number	Proportion of all deaths (per cent)
1	74	31	41.9
2	46	14	30.4
3	20	9	45.0
4	7	—	—
5–10	10	4	40.0
All	157	58	36.9

* For definition of parity see page 8

Women booked for delivery in private nursing homes

One woman only was booked for delivery in a private nursing home. She was a non-resident patient from Kuwait who was transferred to the United Kingdom during her pregnancy and died from acute myelomonocytic leukaemia on the day of her delivery at 30 weeks gestation.

Women booked for delivery in hospitals of the armed services

Two women who were booked for delivery in armed services hospitals are included in the series. One primigravida aged 19 was transferred to a teaching hospital when a diagnosis of acute myeloid leukaemia was made. She died about six weeks after a premature delivery at 35 weeks gestation. The other patient also a primigravida aged 26 was transferred to an NHS hospital with premature rupture of the membranes at 35 weeks. She collapsed during labour as the result of a pulmonary embolism and died following an emergency Caesarean section.

Women booked for consultant units

Two hundred and eighty women (65.6% of all the deaths) were initially booked for delivery in consultant units. A further 2 women from home and 15 from general practitioner units had their bookings transferred to consultant units during the course of their pregnancy, making a total of 297. Associated causes were responsible for the deaths of 147 (49.3%) and 150 died from true causes of maternal death. The arrangements for the antenatal care of these 297 women are shown in Table 16.9. It is not known what proportion of all women booked for hospital confinement have shared antenatal care with the general practitioner but it is thought to be of the same order as that shown for the women who died. (See Table 16.9).

Table 16.9: *Arrangements for antenatal care of women booked for delivery in consultant unit, 1976 – 78*

	Number of Cases	
	True maternal deaths	Associated maternal deaths
Hospital consultant(s) only	37	38
'Shared' care	112	105
GP and midwife only	1	3
Not stated	–	1
	150	147

The age and parity distribution of the 297 women who died are shown in Tables 16.10 and 16.11, and the proportion with avoidable factors. Data on the overall booking arrangements for those women who were delivered in consultant units during the triennium, but who did not die are not available and therefore an accurate death rate cannot be calculated. The number initially booked are not sufficiently comparable with the number finally delivered for this figure to be used.

Table 16.10: *The number of deaths of women by age, booked for delivery in consultant units, and the proportion with avoidable factors, 1976 – 78*

Age	All deaths Number	Deaths with avoidable factors as percentage of all deaths
< 19	16	31.2
20 – 24	64	31.2
25 – 29	109	38.5
30 – 34	68	30.9
35 – 39	26	34.6
40 – 44	11	72.7
45 +	3	33.3
All	297	35.7

Table 16.11: *The number of deaths of women by parity* booked for delivery in consultant units, and the proportion with avoidable factors 1976 – 78*

Parity	All deaths Number	Deaths with avoidable factors as percentage of all deaths
1	135	37.0
2	67	20.9
3	52	32.7
4	23	52.2
5 – 9	19	63.2
10 +	1	100.0
All	297	35.7

* For definition of parity see page 8

Deaths before 28 weeks

Eighteen of the 297 women died before the 28th week of pregnancy, 5 from true causes and 13 from associated causes of maternal death.

Table 16.12: *Place of death of women who died before 28th week of pregnancy booked for consultant units*

Place of death	True deaths			Associated deaths		
	Total	Unavoidable	Avoidable	Total	Unavoidable	Avoidable
Obstetric consultant unit	1	—	1	—	—	—
Other consultant unit	2	2	—	6	5	1
Intensive care unit	—	—	—	5	2	3
At home	2	1	1	2	1	1
Total	5	3	2	13	8	5

In the 5 true deaths an avoidable factor was present in 2 cases. One patient who had a previous myomectomy operation died at home as the result of a ruptured uterus. Two died following spontaneous abortion, one from pulmonary embolism and the other from anaesthetic complications. Another woman died from pulmonary embolism at 21 weeks of pregnancy. The fifth patient died suddeny at home at 11 weeks of pregnancy and no cause was established despite a post-mortem examination.

In the 13 associated deaths avoidable factors were present in 5 cases. In one case of a diabetic patient the antenatal care was considered to have been inadequate and there was also delay in diagnosing an underlying bronchopneumonia. One patient, a known drug addict, died following an overdose of drugs at fourteen weeks of pregnancy. Another woman who died as the result of an adrenal crisis had possibly not been taking her medication regularly. The other two cases were associated with spontaneous abortions at 22 and 26 weeks respectively. (Table 16.12).

Deaths at 28 weeks or over (died undelivered)

Thirty eight of the women died undelivered after the 28th week of pregnancy, 18 from true maternal causes and 20 from associated causes, Table 16.13. They had all been initially booked for a consultant unit. Only 3 of the 20 associated deaths were judged to have an avoidable factor. One patient aged 36 years with pre-existing hypertension was a very poor attender at the antenatal clinic and took her own discharge 2 days after admission to hospital at 31 weeks of pregnancy. She died at home the following week from coronary thrombosis. The other two patients died as the result of haemorrhage from arterial aneurysms, one of the hepatic artery and the other associated with abnormal renal arteries. (See Chapter 14).

Table 16.13: *Place of death of women who died after 28th week of pregnancy (undelivered) booked for consultant units*

Place of death	True deaths			Associated deaths		
	Total	Unavoidable	Avoidable	Total	Unavoidable	Avoidable
Obstetric consultant unit	11	6	5	7	4	3
Other consultant unit	3	2	1	1	1	—
Intensive care unit	—	—	—	4	4	—
At home	3	1	2	7	7	—
Other (in ambulance etc)	1	—	1	1	1	—
Total	18	9	9	20	17	3

In the 18 true deaths, at least one avoidable factor was present in 8 and in 5 of these it was related to inadequate antenatal care. One patient, para 9, aged 42 years with essential hypertension refused admission to hospital. She died at home as the result of haemorrhage from placental abruption at about 33 weeks of pregnancy. Three of the women died from pulmonary embolism, one at home and two in hospital. In all these cases it was felt that the doctors concerned with their care had failed to take adequate action when the first symptoms appeared. The other patient died from fulminating pre-eclampsia. Three of the 18 women died at home one from spontaneous rupture of the uterus at 29 weeks gestation, and the other two, among those already mentioned, from haemorrhage and pulmonary embolism respectively. The causes of death in these 18 women, all true maternal deaths are shown in Table 16.14.

Table 16.14: *Causes of true maternal deaths at 28th week of pregnancy and after of women booked at consultant units who died undelivered 1976–78*

ICD Code	Causes	Number of cases
633	Ectopic pregnancy	1
641	Antepartum haemorrhage	2
642	Hypertension complicating pregnancy	1
643	Excessive vomiting in pregnancy	1
646	Other complications of pregnancy	1
665	Other obstetrical trauma	1
668	Complications of the administration of anaesthetic or other sedation in labour and delivery	2
669	Other complications of labour and delivery	1
673	Obstetrical pulmonary embolism	8
Total		18

Deaths at 28 weeks or over (died after delivery)

Two hundred and forty one of the 297 died after the delivery of an infant of 28 weeks or more, 127 from true causes and 114 from associated causes (Table 16.15).

Table 16.15: *Deaths during and after the 28th week (delivered) of women booked for consultant units 1976–78*

Booking	True deaths			Associated deaths		
	Total	Unavoidable	Avoidable	Total	Unavoidable	Avoidable
Initially for consultant unit	121	48	73	104	94	10
Booking transferred from home	1	1	—	1	1	—
Booking transferred from general practitioner unit	5	2	3	9	7	2
Total	127	51	76	114	102	12

In the 114 associated cases an avoidable factor was present in 12 cases and in 5 of the 12 this was present in the antenatal period. In 2 cases avoidable factors were attributed to the patients. One asthmatic patient refused to accept medication before or after delivery and died at home from an acute attack 17 days after delivery. Another patient with an ureteric calculus refused operation during pregnancy and following recurrent urinary tract infections died from chronic renal failure 5 months after delivery. Two other patients one with

Table 16.16: *Place of death of women who died during and after the 28th week of pregnancy (delivered) booked for consultant unit 1976–78 compared with 1973–75, and the number with avoidable factors*

Place of Death	1973–75						1976–78					
	True deaths			Associated deaths			True deaths			Associated deaths		
	Total	Unavoidable	Avoidable	Total	Unavoidable	Avoidable	Total	Unavoidable	Avoidable	Total	Unavoidable	Avoidable
Obstetric consultant unit	66	24	42	22	20	2	54	16	38	12	12	—
Other consultant unit	15	6	9	32	26	6	17	9	8	39	37	2
Intensive care unit	41	14	27	13	9	4	42	16	26	25	18	4
At home	7	7	—	14	13	1	12	9	3	22	20	2
Other	4	3	1	6	5	1	2	1	1	16	15	1
Total	133	54	79	87	73	14	127	51	76	114	102	12

temporal lobe epilepsy and one with ulcerative colitis had originally been unsuitably booked for delivery in general practitioner units. In the 127 true maternal deaths an avoidable factor was present in 76 cases, but in only 24 was the antenatal period involved.

In 10 of the 24 cases the patient herself was at fault because of non-attendance for antenatal care until after the 20th week of pregnancy, for defaulting from the antenatal clinic or for refusing to enter hospital for treatment despite medical advice. Four of the women later developed hypertensive diseases of pregnancy, as did 6 other patients whose poor antenatal care was the responsibility of their general practitioners or the consultant unit staff. In the cases of one primigravida and of two women with twin pregnancies administrative failure to provide adequate supporting services at small units was at least partly responsible for disasters. Postpartum haemorrhage occurred in all 3 cases and in two instances blood had to be obtained from a considerable distance. In one of the cases of twin pregnancy no paediatric assistance was available and haemorrhage occurred when the obstetrician had to leave the mother to attempt to resuscitate the babies.

Of the 127 true deaths following delivery after 28 weeks of pregnancy 42 women died following transfer to intensive care units and 17 to other specialized units such as neurosurgical or renal units. This is indicative of the efforts made to secure optimum treatment for the patients following obstetric complications. The numbers involved are very similar to those in 1973−75 triennium (Table 16.16).

The causes of death in these 127 women are listed in Table 16.17.

Table 16.17: *Causes of true maternal deaths at 28th week of pregnancy and after of women booked in consultant units who died after delivery 1976−78*

ICD Code	Cause	Number of Cases
641	Antepartum haemorrhage, abruptio placentae and placenta praevia	5
642	Hypertension complicating pregnancy, childbirth and the puerperium	20
646	Other complications of pregnancy	7
665	Other obstetrical trauma	12
666	Postpartum haemorrhage	14
668	Complications of the administration of anaesthetic or other sedation in labour and delivery	19
669	Other complications of labour and delivery	1
670	Major puerperal infection	11
673	Obstetrical pulmonary embolism	32
674	Other and unspecified complications of the puerperium	6
Total		127

The outcome for the baby—booked and unbooked in consultant units

Of the 297 women booked for consultant units either initially or during the course of their pregnancy, 279 died after the 28th week of pregnancy. Of these 279 women, 38 died undelivered, in 32 cases the fetus being lost with the mother. Six women were delivered by post-mortem Caesarean section, resulting in 2 live births, both babies dying in the early neonatal period, and 4 stillbirths. Two hundred and forty-one women were delivered before death, including 7 with a twin pregnancy; 208 babies were born alive with 10 early neonatal deaths and 40 were stillborn. The total fetal loss after the 28th week of pregnancy in women who died having been booked for confinement in consultant units was therefore 88 out of 286 (30.8%).

A total of 26 women who were 28 weeks pregnant or more, were admitted to consultant units as unbooked emergencies. Seven had made no arrangements for delivery and 19 were unbooked for delivery in general practitioner units. Two of the women died undelivered, the fetus in each case being lost with the mother. Twenty-four women were delivered before death; 17 babies were born alive with 3 early neonatal deaths and 7 were stillborn. The fetal loss after the 28th week of pregnancy in unbooked cases was 12 (46%) some 15.2% higher than in the women who had been booked.

Booking arrangements by Social Class

The women in the enquiry who died from true obstetric causes have been classified into social classes using the 1970 'Classification of Occupations' (OPCS, 1970).

Table 16.18 analyses the booking arrangements of the 194 who died where the social class and booking arrangements were both known, and where the duration of pregnancy at the time of death was more than 12 weeks. [Of the patients with no booking arrangements where no duration of pregnancy was stated, who died from true obstetric causes, the 8 who died from ectopic pregnancy, or from anaesthesia associated with an operation for ectopic pregnancy, have been excluded, but the 2 patients who died from haemorrhage and puerperal sepsis respectively have been included as their deaths were obviously after the 12th week of pregnancy.]

Table 16.18: *Booking arrangements by social class: true maternal deaths after the 12th week of pregnancy 1976–78*

Social class	Total	Booking Arrangements				
		No booking	Home	General practitioner unit	Consultant unit	Service hospital
I	22	1	—	2	19	—
II	28	2	1	3	22	—
III	74	10	2	9	53	—
IV	41	8	1	3	29	—
V	12	4	—	1	7	—
Others	17	2	—	—	14	1

Reference

Office of Population, Censuses and Surveys, 1970. *Classification of occupations, 1970*, London, HMSO.

17. Factors influencing maternal mortality in the series of reports from 1952 to 1978

The series of confidential enquiries into maternal deaths began in 1952. The present report is the ninth of the 3-yearly reports in which the findings have been published. Table 17.1 shows the numbers of maternal deaths, included in each of the 9 triennial reports divided into true obstetric deaths, and associated deaths.

Table 17.1: *Total deaths in the 9 enquiry series compared with total maternities, England and Wales 1952–1978*

Triennial Report	Total maternities in England and Wales	Deaths in the Enquiry directly due to pregnancy and childbirth (including abortion)		Deaths in the Enquiry associated with pregnancy and childbirth	
		Number	Rate per million maternities	Number	Rate per million maternities
1952–54	2,052,953	1094	523.9	316	153.9
1955–57	2,113,471	861	407.4	339	160.4
1958–60	2,294,414	742	323.4	254	110.7
1961–63	2,520,420	692	274.6	244	96.8
1964–66	2,600,367	579	222.7	176	67.7
1967–69	2,457,444	455	185.2	243	98.9
1970–72	2,298,198	355	154.5	251	109.2
1973–75	1,921,569	235	122.3	155	80.7
1976–78	1,748,849	227	129.8	200	113.8

There has continued to be an increase in the percentage of known maternal deaths covered in the enquiry series, and in this report this has reached over 99% of the known true obstetric deaths compared with 93% in the previous triennium. Thus, although compared with the 1973–75 series there has only been a very small decrease in the number, from 235 to 227, of true obstetric deaths reported to the Enquiry, the actual fall was greater, probably from 254 to 228, if the true deaths from each triennium known to the Registrar General but not reported to the Enquiry are taken into account. Combined with a continuing fall in the birth rate, which reached its lowest level in 1977, this has resulted in the estimated death rate per million maternities remaining virtually unchanged at 132.2 per million in 1973–75 to 130.4 per million in 1976–78.

This is in contrast with the fall in rate between the 1970–72 and 1973–75 triennia.

	True deaths reported to the Enquiry		Corrected true deaths, including unreported known true deaths	
	Number	Rate per million maternities	Number	Rate per million maternities
1970–72	355	154.5	387	168.4
1973–75	235	122.3	254	132.2
1976–78	227	129.8	228	130.4

On the same basis the estimated death rate for the true deaths for each of the 3 years in the triennium, per million maternities was:-

1976 (81 deaths)   138.6
1977 (76 deaths)   133.6
1978 (71 deaths)   119.2 (including the one unreported true death)

It is apparent that the corrected maternal death rate in 1976–78 is little different from that in 1973–75. One of the reasons for the lack of further improvement is probably the factor mentioned in the 1973-75 Report that a decrease in the size of families has led to a relative increase of first births in which the mothers are more at risk. Other compensating changes have also occurred which would tend to reduce the mortality rate, namely an increase in the proportion of women having second babies, who are at relatively low risk and a decrease in those having fifth or subsequent babies who are at greater risk.

The number of deaths from associated causes rose again in the present report from 155 in 1973–75 to 200. It is always difficult to be sure of the reasons for the fluctuation in the number of associated deaths reported to the Enquiry. MCW 97 reports were received for all the deaths identified by the Registrar General as being from associated causes but it has always been recognized that these are unlikely to cover all those deaths which would come within the wide definition used in the Enquiry of death occurring within 1 year of pregnancy or childbirth. An associated death may not be identifiable from the death certificate alone as it requires only that causes considered to be directly responsible for, or contributory to death are entered, and it is possible that pregnancy will not be recorded, particularly if it occurred some time before death.

Associated deaths are discussed in Chapter 14. As already mentioned and defined in that Chapter and in Chapter 1* of this report these deaths have been further divided into indirect maternal deaths and fortuitous deaths. Seventy-six deaths have been classified in Chapter 14 as indirect deaths as have the 21 deaths from cardiac disease which are included in Chapter 6, making a total of

* see page 7

97 indirect maternal deaths. One hundred and three deaths have been classified as fortuitous. Despite careful consideration of the individual cases it was not always easy to decide how deaths from some of the associated causes should be placed in the different classifications. For example out of 24 deaths from intracranial haemorrhage, some of which occurred during pregnancy and the puerperium, it was decided that only one was an indirect maternal death and that the others were unrelated to pregnancy. Similarly out of 33 deaths from neoplastic disease, only 8 were judged to be indirect maternal deaths.

In this 1976–78 series the 4 main causes of maternal death, with the 1973–75 figures in brackets were pulmonary embolism 45 (35) hypertensive diseases of pregnancy 29 (39) uterine haemorrhage 26 (21) and sepsis 24 (28); ectopic pregnancy with 21 (21) deaths was in fifth position. For the first time since the series began in 1952, abortion 14 (29) was not among the first 4 main causes of maternal death, see Table 17.2. The number of deaths due to abortion, ectopic pregnancy and anaesthesia will be found to be different from those in Tables 1.9 and 1.10 in Chapter 1, this is because in Table 17.2 *all* the deaths associated with anaesthesia have been classified to this cause and not to the indication for operation.

Table 17.2: *Causes of true maternal deaths (ie directly due to pregnancy or childbirth) 1970–78*

Numbers of deaths (Rates per million maternities)			Excluded under International definition	
1970–72	1973–75	1976–78	1976–78	
61 26.5	35 18.2	45 25.7	2	Pulmonary embolism
30 13.1	22 11.4	30 17.2	2	Anaesthesia, including deaths associated with operations, for abortion and ectopic pregnancy
47 20.5	39 20.3	29 16.6	—	Hypertensive diseases of pregnancy
27 11.7	21 10.9	26 14.9	1	Haemorrhage
34 14.8	19 9.9	21 12.0	—	Ectopic pregnancy
32 13.9	22 11.4	17 9.7	2	Sepsis, excluding abortion
74 32.2	27 14.0	14 8.0	1	Abortions
12 5.2	11 5.7	14 8.0	—	Ruptured uterus
22 9.6	14 7.3	11 6.3	—	Amniotic fluid embolism
16 7.0	25 13.0	20 11.4	1	Other causes
335 154.5	235 122.3	227 129.8	9	Total

In the present report the number of deaths directly due to uterine haemorrhage was 26, an increase from 21 in the previous report. This was due to an increase in the number of deaths from postpartum haemorrhage at 17, the highest number since the 1964–66 triennium. The death rate per million maternities rose from 10.9 in 1973–75 to 14.9 in 1976–78. There were 14 other deaths in which antepartum and postpartum haemorrhage contributed to the deaths. There were also 21 deaths from haemorrhage associated with ectopic pregnancy, 14 with rupture of the uterus and one with spontaneous abortion. Haemorrhage from all causes remained a major factor occurring in 76 (33.5%) of the 227 true maternal deaths in the series.

The number of deaths from hypertensive diseases of pregnancy fell from 39 in 1973–75 to 29 in 1976–78, and the death rate per million maternities also fell from 20.3 in 1973–75 to 16.6 in 1976–78. This was the first real improvement in the death rate since the 1967–69 series (Table 2.1). The numbers of deaths from pre-eclampsia fell only slightly from 18 to 16, but those from eclampsia fell from 21 in 1973–75 to 13 in 1976–78. All the deaths from eclampsia and pre-eclampsia were judged to be due to a complication directly due to the condition.

For the first time in the series of reports, pulmonary embolism was the most frequent cause of death from true obstetric causes at 45 compared with 35 in 1973–75. The death rate per million maternities also rose from 19.8 in 1973–75 to 26.9 in 1976–78, when the deaths from pulmonary embolism following abortion, 3 in 1973–75 and 2 in 1976–78 are also included. The increase in deaths from pulmonary embolism was in deaths following delivery, 32 in 1976–78 compared with 21 in 1973–75, and these were mainly in women under 30 years of age. The number of deaths from pulmonary embolism in pregnancy was 13, one less than in the previous triennium. Eight of the 13 deaths during pregnancy were sudden and unexpected. In 13 of the other 32 deaths which followed Caesarean section and vaginal delivery there were warning signs and symptoms of thromboembolism and it is in the earlier recognition of these, followed by effective treatment, that hope for a reduction in deaths from this cause must lie.

The number of deaths from sepsis fell from 28 in 1973–75 to 24 in 1976–78, and there was a small decrease in the death rate per million maternities from 14.6 to 13.7 in the same period. Deaths from sepsis after abortion at 7 remained virtually unchanged at the low level reached in the previous triennium. Four of the deaths from sepsis following surgical procedures were due to perforation of the bowel. If abdominal complications occur after delivery there should be early consultation with a general surgeon and if need be with a microbiologist and greater readiness to open the abdomen.

The deaths from ectopic pregnancy were the same in number at 21, as in the previous triennium. The main hazards of ectopic pregnancy reside in the difficulty in diagnosis and delay in operating.

For the first time since the beginning of the series, deaths due to abortion were not in the first 4 main causes of maternal death and abortion is now in seventh position. There were only 14 deaths from all types of abortion of which 8 followed legal abortions. There was a small reduction in the total number of legal abortions performed during 1976–78, 404,235 compared with

469,791 in 1973—75. There were only 4 deaths in the triennium from illegal abortion. This is a remarkable reduction when compared with the triennium 1964—1966 the last complete triennium before the Abortion Act came into force in April 1968, when there were 98 deaths from this cause.

The number of deaths directly associated with anaesthesia was 30 and in another 10 cases anaesthesia was considered to have contributed to the morbidity which lead to death. This compares with 31 deaths directly associated with anaesthesia and 6 contributory deaths in 1973—75. There was again no accurate information available about the total number of anaesthetics given to obstetric patients during the period 1976—78 and so it was not possible to calculate a death rate based on the incidence of anaesthesia. However, the incidence associated with anaesthesia per million maternities showed a slight rise to 17.2, compared with 16.1 in the previous two triennia. The percentage of deaths associated with anaesthesia among true maternal deaths was 13.2 the same as in 1973—75.

In this triennium there were 21 deaths from associated cardiac disease, almost the same as 1973—75, when 20 such deaths occurred. Eighteen of these deaths were from acquired cardiac disease and only 3 from congenital cardiac disease. Seven of the deaths from acquired cardiac disease were from coronary artery disease, compared with 3 from rheumatic heart disease.

Booking arrangements

There were 84 women who had made no booking arrangements (Table 16.4). The proportion of births taking place at home was even smaller than in the previous triennium (Table 16.3)—2% compared with 4.5% in 1973—75. In this series there were only 6 deaths among women initially booked for home confinement and 2 of these had their booking transferred to a consultant unit during the course of their pregnancy.

As previously described in Chapter 16 an attempt was made in this report to divide the general practitioner units into 'separate' and 'other' units depending upon their distance from consultant obstetric units and other supporting services. There were 52 deaths among women initially booked for confinement in a general practitioner unit and 13 of these were booked for 'separate' units. (Table 16.5 and 16.6). In the absence of reliable information concerning the total number of women who were initially booked for delivery in general practitioner units during the triennium, it is not possible to work out a separate death rate for those women booked for general practitioner units.

Similarly it is not possible, on present available data, to separate the total number of women booked for hospital confinement into those booked for consultant units and general practitioner units, where both types of unit are situated on the same premises. Therefore no separate death rate for those 280 women initially booked in consultant units can be calculated.

In some cases both the 'separate' general practitioner units and small consultant units, isolated from the full facilities of a district general hospital, were in difficulties due to shortages of experienced obstetric, paediatric and anaesthetic staff and of pathological services, especially for blood transfusions. It is unwise for any obstetric patients, but particularly those judged to be at high risk, to be booked for delivery except where full general hospital facilities are available.

Age and parity

Deaths and mortality rates analysed by age and parity of the women in the enquiry series, who died from true obstetric causes are shown in Appendix A, Tables A2 and A3. These show that the risks were higher for first births than for second ones for all age groups, and higher than for third births under the age of 25 years. Between 25 and 29 years the risks for first and third births were similar, but over 30 years the risk for third births were rather higher until the age of 40 years when there was a steep rise in the risk for first births. The rates for second births between 35 and 39 and fourth births between 30 and 39 years were unusually low, but the relatively lower rates for the highest parity women under 40 years, observed in the 1973–75 triennium, were not evident. Under the age of 20 years risks were greater for first and second births than in the 20–24 year age group.

Marital status

The marital status of the 427 women included in the 1976–78 enquiry is shown in Table 17.3. During 1976–78 the average annual percentage of illegitimate live births was 9.7. It is not known how many of the pregnancies in the 3.5% of deaths which occured in the widowed, divorced and separated were illegitimate, but some would certainly have been so. The proportion of maternal deaths in known illegitimate pregnancies in the enquiry series 8.9% was slightly lower than the proportion of illegitimate births in the maternity population as a whole.

Table 17.3: *Marital status in relation to maternal deaths 1976–78*

Marital Status	True Deaths	Associated Deaths	Total	Percentage of series
Married	194	180	374	87.6
Single	33	16	38	8.9
Widowed	3	—	3	
Divorced	5	2	7	3.5
Separated	3	2	5	
Total	227	200	427	100

Table 17.4: *Live births* occurring in England and Wales to women born outside the United Kingdom [compared with those to women born in the United Kingdom]*

Country of origin of mother	1976		1977		1978	
	Number of births in thousands	Percentage of all live births	Number of births in thousands	Percentage of all live births	Number of births in thousands	Percentage of all live births
Irish Republic	11.4	2.0	10.4	1.8	9.8	1.6
Old Commonwealth	2.1	0.4	2.2	0.4	2.2	0.4
New Commonwealth	33.9	5.8	34.8	6.1	36.8	6.2
Pakistan	8.2	1.4	9.5	1.7	11.2	1.9
Other foreign countries	16.9	2.9	17.3	3.0	18.2	3.0
Total outside United Kingdom	72.4	12.4	74.2	13.0	78.1	13.1
In United Kingdom	511.2	87.5	494.5	86.9	517.8	86.8
Not stated	0.7	0.1	0.6	0.1	0.5	0.1
Total	584.3	100.0	569.3	100.0	596.4	100.0

* The correction used elsewhere for 'maternities' is not available for the data about country of origin of the parents.

Country of origin

The country of origin is known for all but one of the 227 women who died from true obstetric causes included in the 1976–78 enquiry, 44 of whom came from the New Commonwealth (and Pakistan). Table 17.4 shows the percentage of live births in England and Wales, occurring to women born outside the United Kingdom. On the assumption that the proportion of total births is not significantly different from the proportion of live births to women from the New Commonwealth (and Pakistan) then of the 1,766,169 total births to all women in 1976–78, 135,642 were to such women. The maternal mortality in these women was 0.32 per 1000 total births, and for all other women in the series 0.11.

Of the 200 women who died from associated causes 28 (14%) were known to have been born in the New Commonwealth (and Pakistan), 8 (14%) in foreign countries and the remaining 164 in the United Kingdom or Eire. The maternal mortality from associated causes was almost double for the New Commonwealth group of mothers being 0.21 per 1000 total births for the New Commonwealth (and Pakistan) and 0.11 for all the others.

Social class

The women in the enquiry series who died from true and associated causes have been classified into social classes (see Table 1.3, page 2). Table 17.5 shows the number of deaths of women for each social class by true and associated causes and whether there were avoidable factors.

Table 17.5: *Numbers of deaths by social class, whether true or associated, and whether there were avoidable factors in England and Wales, 1976 – 78*

Social Class	Number of true maternal deaths		Number of associated maternal deaths			
	With avoidable factors	Without avoidable factors	With avoidable factors		Without avoidable factors	
			All	"Indirect" deaths	All	"Indirect" deaths
I	11	11	—	—	20	8
II	17	14	2	2	24	10
III	54	41	16	12	76	33
IV	25	20	5	2	27	14
V	10	3	—	—	5	1
Others	14	7	6	5	19	10

The distribution by social class of all true and associated deaths is very similar to that for legitimate births. See Table 1.3.

In the triennium a total of 54 avoidable factors were attributed to patients, and these were distributed between 38 individual women. The distribution by social class of these women, when compared with the distribution of all legitimate births, showed as might be expected an increased proportion in Social Classes IV and V and also among those where the social class was not stated. This latter group included those women whose social class could not readily be determined as they or their husbands were unemployed or there was insufficient information available. The exclusion of illegitimate births, however, probably affected this comparison.

Avoidable factors

The number of deaths in which avoidable factors were considered to be present is shown for each cause of death in Appendix A, Table A1, and these factors have been discussed in the corresponding chapters.

Of the 227 deaths directly due to pregnancy or childbirth which are included in the present report 132 (58.1%) had one or more avoidable factors. Of the 200 deaths associated with, but not directly due to pregnancy or childbirth an

Table 17.6: *Number of deaths with avoidable factors, 1952 – 78*

	Deaths directly due to pregnancy or childbirth	Deaths associated with pregnancy or childbirth
1952–54	472	53
1955–57	353	57
1958–60	315	45
1961–63	262	34
1964–66	263	23
1967–69	255	36
1970–72	191	49
1973–75	140	25
1976–78	132	29*

* 21 were indirect maternal deaths

Table 17.7: *Deaths with avoidable factors as percentages of deaths 1952–1978*

	1952 –54	1955 –57	1958 –60	1961 –63	1964 –66	1967 –69	1970 –72	1973 –75	1976 –78
Deaths directly due to pregnancy and childbirth	43.1	41.0	42.5	37.9	44.6	56.0	53.8	59.6	58.1
Deaths directly due to pregnancy and childbirth excluding abortion and ectopic pregnancy*	40.0	37.3	38.9	34.4	34.9	49.0	50.0	57.8	59.0
All deaths associated with pregnancy and childbirth	16.8	16.8	17.7	13.9	13.1	14.8	19.5	16.1	14.5
Indirect maternal deaths	—	—	—	—	—	—	—	—	21.6

* Deaths associated with anaesthesia given during the treatment of these conditions have also been excluded.

avoidable factor was present in 29 (14.5%). If the indirect maternal deaths are considered separately there was an avoidable factor present in 21 of the 97 (21.6%) (Tables 17.6 and 17.7).

The presence of an avoidable factor does not mean that death could have been prevented, or that a factor identified as avoidable was the direct cause of the mother's death. However it does imply that there was some departure from the generally accepted standards of satisfactory care during the triennium, which may have contributed to the fatal outcome. The proportion of deaths directly due to pregnancy and childbirth, true obstetric deaths, considered to have an avoidable factor in 1976—78, 58.1% is very similar to that in the previous triennium 1973—75 when it was 59.6%. There is also little difference between the two triennia, when deaths from abortion and ectopic pregnancy are excluded, in 1976—78 59% had avoidable factors compared with 57.8% in 1973—75.

The proportion of associated deaths with avoidable factors was a little lower at 14.5% in 1976—78 compared with 16.1% in 1973—75. The avoidable factors noted in indirect maternal deaths, 21.6% cannot be compared with earlier triennia as this is the first Report in which these deaths have been separately identified.

The apportionment of responsibility for avoidable factors in all the deaths in the Enquiry is shown in Table 17.8. For the purposes of this table the members of the consultant unit obstetric staff have been considered as a whole, and anaesthetists of all grades grouped together.

Table 17.8: *The apportionment of responsibility for and time of occurrence of, avoidable factors in the maternal deaths of the 1976—78 enquiry series. (The numbers in this table are not mutually exclusive)*

Responsible Person	Total	Antenatal period	Labour or operative procedure	Puerperium or post-operative period
	Number %	Number %	Number %	Number %
Patient	54(23.1)	38(36.2)	7(7.8)	9(23.1)
General Practitioner	30(12.8)	21(20.0)	4(4.4)	5(12.8)
Consultant obstetric unit staff	95(40.6)	35(33.3)	43(47.8)	17(43.6)
Midwife	4(1.7)	2(1.9)	2(2.2)	0(0)
Anaesthetist	35(15.0)	3(2.9)	29(32.2)	3(7.7)
Other hospital staff	9(3.8)	4(3.8)	1(1.1)	4(10.3)
Other community staff	1(0.4)	0(0)	0(0)	1(2.6)
Administration	6(2.6)	2(1.9)	4(4.4)	0(0)
Total	234(100.0)	105(100.0)	90(99.9)	39(100.1)

In some of the maternal deaths multiple avoidable factors were present, arising in the antenatal period, during delivery or in the puerperium. Each instance of an avoidable factors has been assigned and recorded in Table 17.8. In the event of doubt about an avoidable factor the death was finally assessed as having no avoidable factors. Out of a total of 234 avoidable factors 105(44.9%) occurred in the antenatal period, 90(38.5%) during labour or an operative procedure and 39(16.7%) in the puerperium or post-operative period.

Avoidable factors associated with antenatal care in true obstetric deaths.

In the antenatal period there were 81 avoidable factors associated with true obstetric deaths.

Twenty eight of the avoidable factors in the antenatal period were attributed to the patient.

In 24 of these 28, avoidable factors were attributed only to the patient herself, in two to the patient and her general practitioner and in two to the patient and the consultant. In 17 of the 28, no booking for delivery had been made, including 6 cases of concealed pregnancy and 4 of illegal abortion. The avoidable factors in the 11 booked cases were mainly associated with failure to attend the antenatal clinic regularly for the recommended antenatal care or in refusing admission to hospital when this was advised.

Eight of the 28 patients to whom avoidable factors were attributed, originated from the New Commonwealth, Pakistan and one from South America. Difficulty with communication was an important factor in most of these cases.

In 17 cases avoidable factors in the antenatal period were attributed to the general practitioner.

In 10 of these 17, avoidable factors were attributed to the general practitioner alone, in 2 to the general practitioner and patient, in one to the general practitioner and midwife, and in 4 to the general practitioner and the consultant. Eight of these patients died as the result of hypertensive diseases of pregnancy. The avoidable factors were mainly delay in referral to a consultant when early signs of pre-eclampsia were evident.

In 27 cases avoidable factors were attributed to the consultant obstetric unit staff.

The cases attributed to the consultant obstetric team included delay in operating on cases of ectopic pregnancy, faulty technique in cases of mid-trimester legal abortion, delay in admission or in starting treatment of hypertensive diseases of pregnancy, and inadequate treatment of antepartum haemorrhage. In one of the latter cases there was also considered to have been an avoidable factor related to administrative mismanagement, when blood had to be obtained from another hospital at a distance of 10 miles, as only 1 unit of Group O Rhesus negative blood was available.

In 2 other cases of ectopic pregnancy which were admitted to general surgical wards, avoidable factors were attributed to general surgeons.

Avoidable factors associated with labour or operative procedures in true obstetric deaths

There was a total of 90 avoidable factors associated with labour or operative procedures.

In 7 instances these were attributed to the patient. These included concealment of pregnancy, refusal to accept treatment and self-induced abortion. General practitioners were involved 4 times in circumstances which included delay in transfer of a patient to the consultant unit and inadequate treatment of sepsis. Twenty nine were attributed to the anaesthetic staff, and in some junior staff had been unable to manage difficult cases, and senior staff were not immediately available to give adequate supervision. Three of these were judged to be particular failures of the administration of the anaesthetic service. In one the anaesthetist had to leave the maternity unit where he had administered an epidural anaesthetic to return to the general hospital. In another, junior staff were unable to deal with a difficult emergency case and when the circumstances were assessed it was judged that inadequate consultant sessions had been provided to give either cover in obstetric emergencies or to train the junior staff properly. In the third instance, involving an isolated maternity unit, there was no one available to assist the anaesthetist when he got into difficulties with the apparatus.

Forty three avoidable factors were attributed to the consultant obstetric unit staff.

There were again some cases where junior obstetric staff were expected to cope with cases beyond their capabilities. On some occasions this was due either to lack of senior staff of appropriate experience to provide adequate supervision, or else to the senior staff having responsibilities for patients in separate units situated over a wide geographical area. *These cases highlight the fact that the labour ward is an intensive care area and that the administrative arrangements in each unit for dealing with unexpected and sudden obstetric catastrophes should be reviewed regularly.*

The 7 other avoidable factors were attributed to the administration, midwives and other staff.

Avoidable factors associated with the puerperium or post-operative period in true obstetric deaths

There were 27 avoidable factors associated with the puerperium or post-operative period.

In 5 these were attributed to the patient. Two patients discharged themselves early after delivery against medical advice and three concealed their pregnancy.

In 3 the general practitioner was involved. In two cases inadequate action was taken when warning symptoms of pulmonary embolism developed; and in the other there was delay in treating an infection following a legal abortion. Fifteen avoidable factors concerned the staff of consultant obstetric units. Most were concerned with inadequate care of cases of haemorrhage or hypertensive disease of pregnancy immediately following delivery, and others involved delay or insufficient treatment of sepsis. As mentioned in previous chapters, earlier consultation with appropriate colleagues might often have improved the outcome.

Avoidable factors were attributed to the anaesthetist in 3 cases in two of which there was inadequate resuscitation following haemorrhage and in one inhalation of stomach contents.

As has been stated in previous reports, clinical management is often a matter of individual judgement, and errors of judgement such as a failure to diagnose a case of ectopic pregnancy or the withholding of anticoagulant drugs in the prevention or treatment of thromboembolic disease have not been assessed as avoidable. However, the assessors have drawn attention to faults of clinical management where these have fallen below a recognized standard, such as failure to institute treatment in early pre-eclampsia, failure to control haemorrhage or delegation of difficult cases to junior staff where experienced help was or should have been present.

The obstetric emergency flying squad

The obstetric emergency flying squad was called out to 4 of the women whose deaths are covered by the Enquiry. The reasons for the calls were as follows:—

Spontaneous abortion (20 weeks gestation)	1 case
Antepartum haemorrhage	2 cases
Air embolism in labour	1 case

These cases are described in the appropriate chapters.

On 2 occasions there was some delay in the arrival of the flying squad but this was not thought to have directly affected the outcome in these specific cases. There was no case where failure to summon the flying squad was thought to have been an avoidable factor.

Family planning, sterilization and termination of pregnancy

The individual case reports in the series do not often record whether a woman failed to seek contraceptive advice, or failed to take it when it had been given, or whether a pregnancy occurred during the use of an unreliable method of contraception, or when a reliable method was not used properly. Of the 227 true deaths covered in the 1976—78 series only 12 (5.3%) were associated with legal or illegal abortion compared with 24 deaths (10.2%) in the 1973—75 series. However this was not likely to have been due to more effective use of contraception, causing a decrease in the number of unwanted pregnancies as measured by the number of legal abortions performed during the triennium but rather reflected the greater availability of legal abortion and safer methods of inducing abortion.

Procedures for sterilization and termination of pregnancy are not without risk to the patient, and the same is true for the contraceptive pill. However, it should now be regarded as an inherent part of modern practice to ensure that as far as possible, a reliable method of contraception or least hazardous method of sterilization is available to a woman when a further pregnancy might affect her health or even put her life at risk.

Appendix A
Tables

Table A1: *Deaths due to or associated with pregnancy and childbirth 1976 – 78*

ICD No	Cause of Death	1976 Total	1976 Avoidable factors pre
I.	**Infective and Parasitic diseases**		
008	Intestinal infections due to other organisms	—	—
038	Septicaemia	—	—
052	Chickenpox	1	—
070	Infectious hepatitis	—	—
135	Sarcoidosis	—	—
II.	**Neoplasms**		
150	Malignant neoplasm of oesophagus	—	—
151	Malignant neoplasm of Stomach	1	—
153	Malignant neoplasm of Colon	—	—
155	Malignant neoplasm of Liver and intrahepatic bile ducts	—	—
162	Malignant neoplasm of trachea, bronchus and lung	1	—
172	Malignant melanoma of skin	—	—
174	Malignant neoplasm of female breast	—	—
181	Malignant neoplasm of placenta	—	—
191	Malignant neoplasm of brain	4	—
199	Malignant neoplasm without specification of site	2	—
200	Lymphosarcoma and reticulosarcoma	—	—
204	Lymphoid leukaemia	—	—
205	Myeloid leukaemia	—	—
225	Benign neoplasm of brain and other parts of nervous system	—	—
239	Neoplasm of unspecified nature	—	—
III.	**Endocrine nutritional and metabolic diseases and immunity disorders**		
253	Disorders of pituitary gland and its hypothalamic control	—	—
255	Disorders of adrenal glands	—	—
278	Obesity and other hyperalimentation	—	—
IV.	**Diseases of blood and blood forming organs**		
282	Hereditary haemolytic anaemias	—	—
286	Coagulation defects	—	—
287	Purpura and other haemorrhagic conditions	—	—
V.	**Mental disorders**		
305	Nondependent abuse of drugs	—	—
VI.	**Diseases of the nervous system and sense organs**		
320	Bacterial meningitis	—	—
323	Encephalitis, myelitis and encephalomyelitis	—	—
345	Epilepsy	—	—
VII.	**Diseases of the circulatory system**		
394	Diseases of mitral valve	—	—
410	Acute myocardial infarction	—	—
414	Other forms of chronic ischaemic heart disease	—	—
415	Acute pulmonary heart disease	—	—
421	Acute and subacute endocarditis	—	—

	1977		1978		1976–78		1976–78
Total	Avoidable factors pres.	Total	Avoidable factors pres.	Total	Avoidable factors pres.	OPCS Code
1	—	—	—	1	—	—
—	—	1	—	1	—	—
1	—	—	—	2	—	1
—	—	—	—	—	—	1
—	—	—	—	—	—	1
1	—	1	1	2	1	2
1	—	1	—	3	—	3
3	—	—	—	3	—	3
—	—	2	—	2	—	2
—	—	—	—	1	—	1
—	—	2	—	2	—	4
—	—	—	—	—	—	1
—	—	1	—	1	—	2
3	—	2	1	9	1	5
—	—	—	—	2	—	2
—	—	—	—	—	—	1
—	—	1	—	1	—	1
—	—	—	—	—	—	3
1	—	—	—	1	—	—
—	—	—	—	—	—	1
—	—	—	—	—	—	1
—	—	—	—	—	—	1
—	—	—	—	—	—	1
—	—	—	—	—	—	1
—	—	—	—	—	—	1
—	—	—	—	1	—	—
—	—	—	—	1	—	1
—	—	—	—	1	—	1
—	—	1	—	2	—	2
—	—	1	—	2	—	4
—	—	—	—	—	—	1
—	—	—	—	—	—	5
—	—	—	—	—	—	1
—	—	—	—	—	—	4
—	—	—	—	—	—	2

ICD No	Cause of Death	1976 Total	Avoidable factors pres
422	Acute myocarditis	—	—
424	Other diseases of endocardium	—	—
425	Cardiomyopathy	—	—
427	Cardiac dysrhythmias	—	—
428	Heart failure	—	—
429	Ill-defined descriptions and complications of heart disease	—	—
430	Subarachnoid haemorrhage	6	—
431	Intracerebral haemorrhage	3	—
432	Other and unspecified intracranial haemorrhage	1	—
433	Occlusion stenosis of precerebral arteries	—	—
434	Occlusion of cerebral arteries	1	—
435	Transient cerebral ischaemia	—	—
441	Aortic aneurysm	—	—
442	Other aneurysm	—	—
446	Polyarteritis nodosa and allied conditions	—	—
453	Other venous embolism and thrombosis	—	—
VIII.	*Diseases of the respiratory system*		
480	Viral pneumonia	—	—
481	Pneumococcal pneumonia	—	—
482	Other bacterial pneumonia	—	—
485	Bronchopneumonia, organism unspecified	—	—
486	Pneumonia, organism unspecified	—	—
487	Influenza	2	—
493	Asthma	—	—
IX.	*Diseases of the digestive system*		
551	Other hernia of abdominal cavity, with gangrene	—	—
553	Other hernia of abdominal cavity with mention of obstruction or gangrene	—	—
555	Regional enteritis	—	—
556	Idiopathic proctocolitis	1	—
558	Other noninfective gastroenteritis and colitis	—	—
560	Intestinal obstruction without mention of hernia	1	1
569	Other disorders of intestine	—	—
571	Chronic liver disease and cirrhosis	—	—
X.	*Diseases of the genitourinary system*		
582	Chronic glomerulonephritis	1	1
621	Disorders of uterus, not elsewhere classified	—	—
XI.	*Complications of pregnancy, childbirth and the puerperium*		
633	Ectopic pregnancy	7	1
634	Spontaneous abortion	2	1
635	Legally induced abortions	—	—
636	Illegally induced abortions	2	2
637	Unspecified abortion	—	—
639	Complications following abortion and ectopic and molar pregnancies	—	—
641	Antepartum haemorrhage, abruptio placentae and placenta praevia	2	1
642	Hypertension complicating pregnancy, childbirth and the puerperium	13	8
643	Excessive vomiting in pregnancy	—	—
646	Other complications of pregnancy, not elsewhere classified	1	—

1977		1978		1976–78		1976–78
Total	Avoidable factors pres.	Total	Avoidable factors pres.	Total	Avoidable factors pres.	OPCS Code
—	—	—	—	—	—	2
—	—	—	—	—	—	1
—	—	—	—	—	—	1
—	—	—	—	—	—	1
—	—	—	—	—	—	3
—	—	—	—	—	—	1
4	—	3	—	13	—	9
1	—	4	—	8	—	5
1	—	—	—	2	—	—
—	—	—	—	—	—	1
—	—	—	—	1	—	2
—	—	—	—	—	—	1
—	—	—	—	—	—	1
—	—	—	—	—	—	1
—	—	—	—	—	—	1
—	—	—	—	—	—	1
—	—	1	—	1	—	—
—	—	—	—	—	—	3
2	1	—	—	2	1	2
—	—	—	—	—	—	2
—	—	—	—	—	—	1
—	—	—	—	2	—	3
—	—	1	—	1	—	3
—	—	—	—	—	—	1
—	—	—	—	—	—	1
—	—	—	—	—	—	1
—	—	—	—	1	—	1
—	—	—	—	2	—	1
—	—	1	1	2	2	1
—	—	—	—	—	—	2
—	—	—	—	—	—	1
—	—	—	—	1	1	1
—	—	—	—	—	—	2
9	4	5	1	21	6	19
—	—	—	—	2	1	3
4	2	4	3	8	5	10
1	1	1	1	4	4	1
—	—	—	—	—	—	2
—	—	1	1	1	1	1
4	2	3	3	9	6	7
7	6	10	8	30	22	39
—	—	2	—	2	—	4
3	1	5	1	9	2	8

ICD No	Cause of Death	1976 Total	Avoidable factors pre
647	Infective and parasitic conditions in the mother classifiable elsewhere but complicating pregnancy, childbirth and puerperium		
.6	Other viral diseases	2	—
.8	Other specified infective and parasitic diseases	1	—
648	Other current conditions in the mother classifiable elsehwere but complicating the pregnancy, childbirth and puerperium		
.0	Diabetes mellitus	2	1
.2	Anaemia	1	—
.4	Mental disorders	5	1
.5	Congenital cardiovascular disorders	1	1
.6	Other cardiovascular diseases	7	2
.7	Bone and joint disorders of back, pelvis and lower limbs	—	—
.9	Other	8	2
653	Disproportion	—	—
654	Abnormality of organs and soft tissues of pelvis	—	—
656	Other fetal and placental problems affecting management of mother	—	—
658	Other problems associated with amniotic cavity and membranes	—	—
659	Other indications for care or intervention related to labour and delivery and not elsewhere classified	—	—
661	Abnormality of forces of labour	—	—
662	Long labour	—	—
663	Umbilical cord complications	—	—
665	Other obstetrical trauma	6	6
666	Postpartum haemorrhage	9	7
668	Complications of the administration of anaesthetic or other sedation in labour and delivery	7	7
669	Other complications of labour and delivery not elsewhere classified	1	1
670	Major puerperal infection	7	4
671	Venous complications in pregnancy and the puerperium	—	—
673	Obstetrical pulmonary embolism	22	8
674	Other and unspecified complications of the puerperium, not elsewhere classified	2	—
XIII.	*Diseases of the musculoskeletal system and connective tissue*		
710	Diffuse diseases of connective tissue	—	—
716	Other and unspecified arthropathies	—	—
737	Curvature of spine	—	—
XV.	*Congenital anomalies*		
745	Bulbus cordis anomalies and anomalies of cardiac septal closure	—	—
747	Other congenital anomalies of circulatory system	—	—
XVI.	*Symptoms, signs and ill-defined conditions*		
780	General symptoms	—	—
799	Other ill-defined and unknown causes of morbidity and mortality	1	—
XVII.	*External causes of injury and poisoning*		
E805	Hit by rolling stock	—	—
E812	Other motor vehicle traffic accident involving collision with another motor vehicle	2	—

	1977		1978		1976–78	1976–78
Total	Avoidable factors pres.	Total	Avoidable factors pres.	Total	Avoidable factors pres.	OPCS Code
—	—	1	—	3	—	2
1	1	1	—	3	—	—
1	—	—	—	3	—	2
1	—	1	—	3	—	3
4	1	6	—	15	2	—
1	1	2	—	4	2	4
7	1	8	1	22	4	3
—	—	1	—	1	—	—
8	3	11	3	37	8	12
—	—	—	—	—	—	2
—	—	—	—	—	—	3
—	—	—	—	—	—	1
—	—	—	—	—	—	1
—	—	—	—	—	—	1
—	—	—	—	—	—	1
—	—	—	—	—	—	6
—	—	—	—	—	—	1
5	4	4	2	15	12	15
3	1	5	4	17	12	12
5	15	8	8	30	30	12
—	—	1	—	2	1	9
6	5	3	2	16	11	8
—	—	1	—	1	—	27
8	8	17	4	57	20	18
6	2	1	—	9	2	13
—	—	—	—	—	—	1
—	—	—	—	—	—	1
—	—	—	—	—	—	1
—	—	—	—	—	—	2
—	—	—	—	—	—	1
—	—	—	—	—	—	1
3	—	—	—	4	—	1
1	—	—	—	1	—	1
2	—	1	—	5	—	5

			1976
ICD No	Cause of Death	Total	Avoidable factors pres
E815	Other motor vehicle traffic accident incolving collision on the highway	1	—
E850	Accidental poisoning by analgesics, antipyretics, antirheumatics	—	—
E854	Accidental poisoning by other psychotropic agents	—	—
E867	Accidental poisoning by gas distributed by pipeline	1	—
E870	Accidental cut, puncture, perforation or haemorrhage during medical care	—	—
E882	Fall from or out of building or other structure	1	—
E890	Conflagration in private dwelling	—	—
E893	Accident caused by ignition of clothing	—	—
E894	Ignition of highly inflammable material	—	—
E901	Excessive cold	—	—
E910	Accidental drowning and submersion	—	—
E912	Inhalation and ingestion of other object causing obstruction of respiratory tract or suffocation	—	—
E938	Other central nervous system depressants	—	—
E950	Suicide and self-inflicted poisoning by solid or liquid substances	—	—
E953	Suicide and self-inflicted injury by hanging strangulation and suffocation	1	—
E957	Suicide and self-inflicted injuries by jumping from a high place	—	—
E958	Suicide and self-inflicted injury by other and unspecified means	1	—
E963	Assault by hanging and strangulation	—	—
E966	Assault by cutting and piercing instrument	1	—
E980	Poisoning by solid or liquid substances, undetermined whether accidentally or purposely inflicted	—	—
E982	Poisoning by other gases, undetermined whether accidentally or purposely inflicted	—	—
E984	Submersion (drowning), undetermined whether accidentally or purposely inflicted	—	—
E987	Falling from high place, undetermined whether accidentally or purposely inflicted	1	—
E988	Injury by other and unspecified means undetermined, whether accidental or purposely inflicted	1	—

	1977		1978		1976–78		1976–78
tal	Avoidable factors pres.	Total	Avoidable factors pres.	Total	Avoidable factors pres.	OPCS Code
—	—	—	—	1	—	1
—	—	—	—	—	—	2
—	—	—	—	—	—	1
—	—	—	—	1	—	1
—	—	—	—	—	—	1
—	—	1	—	2	—	2
—	—	—	—	—	—	1
—	—	—	—	—	—	1
1	—	—	—	1	—	—
—	—	—	—	—	—	1
1	—	—	—	1	—	2
1	—	—	—	1	—	—
—	—	—	—	—	—	1
1	—	2	1	3	1	7
—	—	—	—	1	—	3
—	—	—	—	—	—	1
2	—	—	—	3	—	6
1	—	—	—	1	—	1
—	—	—	—	1	—	1
2	1	—	—	2	1	5
—	—	1	—	1	—	1
1	—	—	—	1	—	1
—	—	1	—	2	—	2
—	—	—	—	1	—	1

Table A2: *Number of deaths by age of mother in the Enquiry 1976–78 compared with those included in 1973–75 and rate per million maternities*

Age (years)	Number of deaths					Rate per million maternities				
	1973–75		1976–78			1973–75		1976–78		
				Associated					Associated	
	'True'	Associated	'True'	All	Indirect	'True'	Associated	'True'	All	Indirect
Under 16	1	–	2	2	1	206.9	–			
16–17	10	6	3	6	5	123.8	84.2	106.3	94.5	65.0
18–19	15	11	13	8	5					
20–24	42	34	38	41	15	67.4	54.6	70.4	76.0	27.8
25–29	63	48	83	71	32	89.4	68.1	130.2	111.3	50.2
30–34	46	35	44	48	26	171.1	130.2	144.9	158.1	85.6
35–39	38	14	22	16	9	408.5	150.5	276.3	200.9	113.0
40–44	17	6	17	7	4	735.1	259.4	975.3	401.6	229.5
45+	3	1	5	1	–	1663.9	554.6	3333.4	666.7	–
Total	235	155	227	200	97	122.3	80.7	129.8	114.4	55.5

Table A3: Number of deaths by parity of mother in the enquiry 1976–78 compared with those included in 1973–75 and rate per million maternities

Parity	Number of deaths					Rate per million maternities				
	1973–75		1976–78			1973–75		1976–78		
	True	Associated	True	Associated		True	Associated	True	Associated	
				All	Indirect				All	Indirect
1	85	55	102	87	46	104.8	67.8	136.6	116.4	61.5
2	55	41	41	54	23	79.5	59.3	63.7	83.9	35.7
3	39	28	36	33	15	151.1	108.5	154.2	141.4	64.3
4	28	10	18	15	7	295.6	105.6	236.1	196.7	91.8
5–9	23	18	27	8	5	378.6	287.7	605.6	188.0	104.4
10 or more	2	1	2	1	–	–	–	–	–	–
Not stated	3	2	1	2	1	–	–	–	–	–
Total	235	155	227	200	97	122.3	80.7	129.8	114.4	55.5

Table A4: *Maternities by age and parity, 1976–1978, England and Wales*

Parity	Age							
	All ages	Under 20	20–24	25–29	30–34	35–39	40–44	45+
All	1,748,851	169,301	539,737	637,683	303,575	79,624	17,431	1,500
1	747,409	136,209	284,199	239,836	71,611	13,164	2,252	138
2	643,922	30,966	198,108	269,285	121,528	20,928	2,967	140
3	233,388	2,008	46,716	91,654	69,697	19,873	3,269	171
4	76,247	106	8,935	26,132	25,845	12,295	2,761	173
5+	47,885	12	1,779	10,776	14,894	13,364	6,182	878

Table A5: *Number of 'true' maternal deaths included in the enquiry 1976–78 by age and parity*

Age (Years)	Parity							
	1	2	3	4	5–9	10+	Not Stated	All
Under 16	2	—	—	—	—	—	—	2
16–17	3	—	—	—	—	—	—	3
18–19	11	2	—	—	—	—	—	13
20–24	31	3	2	2	—	—	—	38
25–29	36	22	14	8	3	—	—	83
30–34	11	12	12	2	7	—	—	44
35–39	4	1	7	3	7	—	—	22
40–44	3	1	1	3	7	2	1	18
45+	1	—	—	—	3	—	—	4
Not stated	—	—	—	—	—	—	—	—
Total	102	41	36	18	27	2	1	227

Table A6: *Death rate of true maternal deaths per million maternities by age and parity 1976–78*

Age (Years)	Parity					
	1	2	3	4	5+	Total
< 20	117.5	64.6	—	—	—	106.3
20–24	109.1	15.1	42.8	233.8	—	70.4
25–29	150.1	81.7	152.7	306.1	278.4	130.2
30–34	153.6	98.7	172.2	77.4	470.0	144.9
35–39	303.9	47.8	352.2	244.0	523.8	276.3
40+ {40–44 / 45+}	673.6	321.9	290.7	1,022.5	1,699.7	1,162.1*
Total	136.5	63.7	154.2	236.1	605.6	129.8*

* *Note* The one death where age was known, but parity was not known has been included in these two totals.

176

Table A7: *Maternities by age and parity, 1970–78, England and Wales*

Parity	Age							
	All ages	Under 20	20–24	25–29	30–34	35–39	40–44	45+
All	5,968,618	620,339	1,988,961	2,075,747	894,884	306,669	76,217	5,801
1	2,481,325	499,284	1,025,348	723,610	180,472	43,461	8,588	552
2	2,095,711	111,862	724,013	858,611	317,613	70,861	12,152	599
3	842,593	8,692	188,616	334,121	221,004	74,950	14,410	800
4	317,585	456	41,718	109,036	101,279	51,692	12,621	783
5+	231,404	45	9,266	50,359	74,516	65,705	28,446	3,067

Table A8: *Estimated number of conceptions, 1970–1978, England and Wales*

Triennia	Age					
	Under 15	15–24	25–34	35–44	45 and over	All ages
1970–72	2,780	1,284,526	1,242,705	246,936	5,157	2,787,368
1973–75	3,640	1,059,419	1,169,762	190,566	4,511	2,432,995
1976–78	3,642	931,252	1,133,552	163,563	4,074	2,241,361

Source: Abortions (642–645)   HIPE
       Ectopic pregnancies   HIPE
       Legal abortions   Series AB and Supplement on abortion
       Maternities   Series FM and Statistical Reviews Pt 11

Appendix B
Maternal deaths reported by
Coroners 1976–78

Since December 1966, after a request to the Secretary of the Coroner's Society of England and Wales, some Coroners have reported to the Chief Medical Officer of the Department of Health and Social Security cases which came to their notice in which a woman was found to be pregnant or recently delivered at the time of death. This has enabled cases to be included in the enquiry series which might otherwise not have been reported. A total of 19 cases relating to maternal deaths occurring in 1976–78 was reported in this way. Sixteen of these 19 cases were matched with a death certificate and a report of a confidential enquiry. The details of these are already incorporated in the relevant sections of this report.

In only 3 cases reported by the Coroners was no confidential enquiry made, nor a matching death certificate found by the Office of Population, Censuses and Surveys. The fact that the death certificate was not traced indicates that the fact of pregnancy did not appear on the death certificate. Therefore, because of the risk of a possible breach of confidentiality these 3 cases were not notified to the regional assessors.

The cause of death in these 3 cases:-

1. Staphylococcal pneumonia
2. Sickle cell disease
3. Suicide (in the puerperium)

All three cases were associated deaths, and were all classified as indirect maternal deaths.

The 3 deaths were reported by cororners in the following regions:-

West Midlands	2
Trent	1

Appendix C
Acknowledgements

This report has been made possible by the help and work of the Area Medical Officers who initiated the enquiries and collected the information, and the consultant obstetricians, anaesthetists and pathologists, general practitioners and midwives who have supplied the detailed case records and the post-mortem reports.

The staff of the Medical Statistics Division of the Office of Population Censuses and Surveys have processed the statistical data and prepared the tables. The authors would like to express their thanks to all these people, and also to the consultant obstetricians and anaesthetists listed below, who have acted as regional assessors and helped in the preparation of this report.

I. *Regional Assessors in Obstetrics*

Northern Region	Professor J K Russell MD FRCOG
Yorkshire Region	Professor J S Scott MD FRCSE FRCOG
Trent Region	Mr Tom Smith MB ChB FRCS FRCOG
East Anglia Region	Mr A P Bentall MA MD DCH FRCOG (until 31.7.78)
	Mr J A Carron Brown FRCS FRCOG (from 1.8.78)
North West Thames Region	Professor J C McClure Browne MS BS BSc FRCS FRCOG (until 31.3.78)
	Mr W G MacGregor FRCS FRCOG (from 1.4.78)
North East Thames Region	Mr G L Bourne FRCS FRCOG
South East Thames Region	Professor Sir Stanley Clayton MD MS FRCS FRCOG (until 31.3.78)
	Mr E D Morris MD FRCS FRCOG (from 1.4.78)
South West Thames Region	Professor Sir John Dewhurst MD ChB FRCS FRCOG
Oxford Region	Mr E A Williams FRCS FRCOG
South Western Region	Mr A Howard John FRCS FRCOG
Wales	Mr J M Bowen BSc MD BCh FRCOG (until 31.7.80)
	Professor B M Hibbard MD FRCOG (from 1.8.80)

179

West Midlands Region
 Sub-Region I   Mr R Logan Edwards FRCS FRCOG
 Sub-Region II   Mr K Baker MD FRCOG
North Western Region   Professor V R Tindall MD FRCS FRCOG
Mersey Region   Mr H H Francis BSc MB ChB FRCS FRCOG
Wessex Region   Professor J K Dennis MB ChB FRCS FRCOG

II. *Regional Assessors in Anaesthesia*

Northern Region   Dr R L McMillan MB ChB FFARCS
Yorkshire Region   Professor D G McDowall MD FFARCS
Trent Region   Professor J A Thornton MD FFARCS
East Anglia Region   Dr Aileen Adams MB ChB FFARCS
North West Thames Region   Dr B A Sellick MB BS FFARCS
                             (until 31.7.78)
                             Professor C M Conway MB FFARCS
                             (from 1.8.78)
North East Thames Region   Dr T Hilary Howells MB ChB FFARCS
South East Thames Region   Dr A H Galley MB BS FFARCS
                             (until 31.8.77)
                             Professor Leo Strunin MD FFARCS
                             (from 1.9.77–31.1.80)
                             Dr J R Nicholson MB FFARCS
                             (from 1.2.80—deceased)
South West Thames Region   Dr H C Churchill-Davidson MA MD FFARCS
Oxford Region   Dr J V Mitchell MA MB MS FFARCS
South Western Region   Dr V Torry Baxter MB ChB FFARCS
                             (deceased)
                             Dr T A Thomas MB ChB FFARCS
                             (from 15.4.78)
Wales   Professor W W Mushin MA FRCS FFARCS
                             (until 14.6.78)
                             Dr Michael Rosen MB ChB FFARCS
                             (from 15.6.78)
West Midlands Region   Professor J S Robinson MD FFARCS
North Western Region   Professor A R Hunter MD FRFPS FRCS
                             FFARCS
Mersey Region   Dr G Jackson Rees MB ChB FFARCS
                             (Until 14.7.78)
                             Dr T H L Bryson MB Chb FFARCS
                             (from 15.7.78)
Wessex   Dr R J Pearce MB BS FFARCS

Printed in England for Her Majesty's Stationery Office
by Hobbs the Printers of Southampton
(1856) Dd718218 C42 11/82 G381